5 STONE, 4 MONTHS, 3 MOUNTAINS

The Learnings & Journal of a Man Finding Wellness, Health, and Fitness at 50

Dave Fernley

Expert Creation Publishing

This book is not intended as a substitute for the medical advice of physicians.
The reader should regularly consult a physician in matters relating to his/
her health and particularly with respect to any symptoms that may require
diagnosis or medical attention.

The information in this book is meant to supplement, not replace, proper
fitness training. Like any sport involving speed, equipment, balance and
environmental factors, fitness training poses some inherent risk. The author
and publisher advise readers to take full responsibility for their safety and
know their limits. Before practicing the skills described in this book, be sure
that your equipment is well maintained, and do not take risks beyond your
level of experience, aptitude, training, and comfort level.

ISBN: 9798687147057

Cover design by: Amanda Walker Fernley

I want to firstly dedicate this book to my wife and business partner, Amanda. We met when I was fit, healthy, and six stone lighter. There was no grey beard trying to hide a fat face in those days. I'd say that I looked 20 years younger than I did when starting off my campaign to get myself fit, slim, and young again. I am sorry for the years I let myself slip. I often wondered if you would have given me a second glance if I had met you more recently. I thank you from the bottom of my heart for being my life partner and best friend. I owe you this campaign to regain health and fitness. Thank you for all your support. I love you dearly.

I also want to thank my kids Jack and Emma. I couldn't be a prouder dad and I can't thank you enough for your support. The past few years have been a topsy-turvy time and as you grow into wonderful young adults, you both fill me with so much pride. You have grown up understanding that all of the long hours and the times away from home, that Amanda and I had to do, was part of our life. You never complained or demanded, you have been wonderful, and I thank you. As you both grow up I hope to share as much of my experiences in business, health, and wealth, and help you on your way to success and happiness.

I have to offer a special note of thanks to my very dear friend Peter Rowan. Peter has been a huge support and inspiration to me during this campaign and I thank him unconditionally. Peter is incredibly modest in his achievements. It is only when you get to know Peter that you find that he is a record holder (held since 1987) for an intense endurance test in the Highlands of Scotland called the Buachaille Dash (won in 4 hours and 48 minutes). Peter has also completed an Ironman Triathlon, and has a wealth of knowledge as a biologist. I sincerely thank you Pete for your support. Long may our friendship continue.

Finally, I want to thank everyone who has supported me over the past few months. There are far too many individuals to mention, but you know who you are. The encouraging comments on social media have been wonderful. The private messages and telephone calls that I have received have been quite humbling. I never set out to inspire other people to get themselves fit and healthy but hearing that I have…is something that I wasn't prepared for.

Thank you everyone.

CONTENTS

FOREWORDS

I first met David at my public speaking event in the October of 2018 in Manchester. Since that day, I have got to know both David and Amanda well as Elite members of my Professional Speakers Academy.

As speakers, experts, mentors, and authorities, we are looked on as leaders in our chosen fields by the people that follow us. This is an honour, but with that honour brings a responsibility to be the very best role model we can be, in all aspects of life including health and wellbeing.

Whilst leading by example as a role model is very important, what is more important is our responsibility to ourselves and our loved ones. Business and life pressures can very easily distract us from looking after our health and fitness. As we get older looking after ourselves has never been more important.

I am honoured to have witnessed how David has transformed his health, both the incredible weight loss result and an exponential increase in fitness. It is those results that now allow him to take on some incredible physical endurance challenges, for example, climbing multiplemountains for charity and now training for marathons and triathlons.

But making such a transformation in life is not easy. You have to have the vision of where you want to be, learn how you are going to realise that vision, formulate the strategy to achieve, take consistent action, re-evaluate, then do it again.

If you are considering such a transformation in your life then reading this book on David's journey is a must for you. This book sets out how David, at the turn of 50 years old, lost five stone in as little as four months, put himself into a position of physical fitness, and is now living a healthy lifestyle to admire and replicate.

I wish David well, and if you are considering your own transformation then I wish you well too.

Andy Harrington
Sunday Times Best Selling Author of 'Passion Into Profit'

◆ ◆ ◆

I met David (and Amanda) two years ago, at one of the Professional Speakers Academy quarterly meetings. We gelled pretty much straight away and have since become very good friends. It now feels like we have known each other for decades!

I was really pleased when David told me back in March that he was going to use the lockdown period as a chance to make substantial changes to his lifestyle. He was nineteen stone and feeling very unfit. By his own admission, he was drinking to excess, eating too much convenience food and snacking between meals. Add to this almost no exercise, and a daily diet of antacid tablets for his chronic indigestion. The writing on the wall was becoming all too visible.

Dave was keen to have a tangible goal to work towards, in terms of weight loss but also in terms of a physical challenge. But his suggestion of completing The National Three Peaks Challenge in under 24 hours took me by surprise. This was a serious physical undertaking and would require not just general fitness, but hill fitness!

He admitted that he'd never been up a mountain in his life before, but had seen this challenge on YouTube and felt sure that it was something he could do once he had lost the weight and regained his fitness! I didn't want to throw cold water on his suggestion but I had serious reservations about him being able to get into a good enough shape in time to do it this Summer. We needed to set a cut off date at the end of July due to available daylight. This was only four months away!!

I knew the only way Dave could lose the necessary weight would be to stick religiously to a training regime on a daily basis and to make big changes to his diet. What were the chances of a 19.2 stone (268lbs, 122kg) guy doing just that and coming out after 4 months not just 5 stone (70lb, 32kg) lighter but fit enough to walk up over 10 000 feet of mountain (at a fair old lick) in under 24 hours with next to no sleep? To be honest, I thought it highly unlikely! But boy, have I enjoyed being proven wrong....

We all do things to avoid a pain or make a gain, and often it's a combination of the two. I'd seen photos of Dave when he was fit and swimming 2 miles a day and understood the overwhelming desire he had to reclaim that body and those days. The pain of being in such poor physical condition gave him the motivation required to make the change.

It's no exaggeration to say that this is one of the most extraordinary transformations I've ever witnessed. It has required an iron will to get out of bed every morning and do the hour walk/run, and to then get on the rower or the weights every afternoon and complete the session. In addition, to knock alcohol on the head completely and be on an intermittent fasting regime to boot!

We did a few training walks to include Scafell Pike, Snowdon and The Yorkshire Three Peaks, and his fitness improved with every outing. Whilst it was great to finally tick the box of The National Three Peaks Challenge, it was not as difficult as The Yorkshire Three Peaks. We had to get up the three hills (about 6000 feet of climb) and walk 24 miles, to be completed in 12 hrs. It was the very hot spell in late May and the temperature was 30°C (86°F).

After 9 hours and two hills completed, Dave was exhausted. In addition, he had a sore back which was causing him a lot of discomfort and he also had chaffed thighs which made every step agony. We ran out of water and I was genuinely worried that he was going to collapse. I said it wasn't important to break the 12 hours but he looked at me and said "I'll do it in under 12 hours if it kills me". That was the moment when I realised he had extraordinary reserves of will power and a huge amount of determination and that The National Three Peaks was a box that he would definitely tick.

A big shout out to his 18 year old son Jack who also completed The Yorkshire Three Peaks and, as I said at the time, although he was similarly exhausted, not once did I hear him moan or ask "How long to go?" A chip off the old block, to be sure!

Dave's fitness journey has also resulted in him taking a serious interest in nutrition and the science behind healthy eating. As he mentions in this book, there is so much nonsense spouted about dietary regimes that gaining a fuller understanding of the science of food has been fundamental to his new eating regime and the subsequent weight loss.

However, I feel that this is just the start of his journey. He has already signed up for a 10k run and a marathon, and is eyeing up a triathlon and an iron man for next year! I have no doubt what-soever that Dave will attain these goals as his mental strength is top drawer and having ticked those boxes in a previous life, going forward I have volunteered to be the driver and/or the drinking partner after the challenges are completed!

Well done mate. You have every reason to be immensely proud of what you've achieved and I look forward to witnessing the next few years....

Peter Rowan

PREFACE

There was no doubt that at the age of 49, over 19 stone (268lbs, 122kg) in weight, and with a resting heart rate of over 85 beats per minute, I was heading for trouble. Add in the stress of business life, and the pressures of standing on stage delivering multi-day presentations to property delegates at various venues throughout the UK. More recently the new threat of COVID-19 has seriously affected business and caused some stress. I had to change my health and lifestyle pretty quick.

I have spent much of my professional life teaching and mentoring business people to develop their property and hospitality businesses which would hopefully provide a better standard of living for themselves and their loved ones. Whilst I love to do that, and whilst I dearly adore my loved ones, it was ironically clear that I was apparently content in thoroughly neglecting myself.

I had been very fit and healthy for years, but I had let a number of difficult times distract and take away the focus that I once had in what was my greatest asset; my body. I came to the realisation that unless I acted quickly there would be a high probability that I would have some form of chronic illness to contend with. The way things were going it was also a fair chance that this might not have been too far away.

However, on 26 March 2020 I set about my transformation which would see me lose 5 stone (70lb, 32kg) in only four short months. My resting heart rate went from over 85bpm down to 59bpm. My fitness slowly returned which would allow me to undertake mountain climbing, hill running, mountain biking, and put myself into a position to confidently register for the Manchester Marathon. I have studied the mind, as well as nutrition, and I have seen huge benefits in intermittent fasting and the effects that this has had on my body.

Whilst I have totally transformed my body, I haven't engaged in any form of fad diet. I haven't had surgery. I haven't bought any weight loss supplements. I haven't weighed or counted food or calories. Neither have I been near a gym (they were all closed down!) but I've had immense fun and I've enjoyed every single meal that I have eaten.

My intention wasn't to write a book when I started my transformation but after the engagement I received on social media, and the inspiring messages and positive conversations that I have had over that period, I decided to journal. It is from that journal, and the education that I sought, that I decided to produce this book, so I really hope you enjoy reading it, and maybe gain some inspiration and ideas too.

CHAPTER 1

UP TO NOW

The Fat Kid At School

I've had a strange relationship with my health, fitness, and weight over the course of my lifetime. As a primary school child, I was one of the fatter kids but I still loved to play sport. I not only played in the school football team, I was the captain. I won plenty of swimming galas and was considered good enough to be picked to swim for the district.

In secondary school I was still one of the fatter kids, until the last couple of years, but in those fatter years I still won annual tennis competitions, played tennis for the school team, played in the football team, did a CSE in Physical Education in which I got a Grade 1, ran cross country, and became the Junior Captain of Stamford Golf Club whilst being a regular in the Golf Club Junior Team.

I believe it is worth noting a very memorable event in my last year in school. I will never forget it and it has been something that I have drawn on in my adult life. We hear people talk about mindset. We hear people talk about focus, determination, and tenacity to achieve as well as gaining desire, clarity, and positivity. The converse to this is fear, worry, overwhelm, insecurity, and negativity.

Mindset and Match

In the July of 1985, I managed to get myself into the final of the school tennis championship. I was up against a guy who I had played before and beaten, so although I was nervous about going into the final I was quietly confident that I could beat him. It was a beautiful summer's day. There wasn't a cloud in the sky and it was hot. The match was to be played at 1pm in the number one court. It was the first court in the row of six and being bigger than the rest of the courts, there was also some room for people to stand and watch, which made it a bit more special.

As I arrived on Court One I was shocked to see an unexpectedly large crowd of people standing around waiting to view the match. As well as the usual and expected school kids, there were teachers spectating too. Immediately my heart started racing with the feeling of self consciousness and dread at playing this match in front of a large crowd. I'd never played tennis in front of a crowd and I had never even considered that I would, despite it being the final. My opponent was already there with a group of his friends. We started the five minute warm up which consisted of knocking the ball backwards and forwards. The confidence that I had previously felt had gone. I was incredibly overawed by the unexpected spectators and painfully self conscious, so I was hitting the ball with a nervousness which meant that I wasn't in flow. As we warmed up I hit the net again and again. We then did some practice serves. Out, out, out, net, out, net, and so it went on. This was awful. This was really awful. My heart was pumping and my arms and legs were feeling like jelly. Five very long and painful minutes went by and it was time to start.

Our PE teacher was the umpire for the match. He tossed a coin for first service, and I lost. My opponent chose me to take the first service. Damn, this isn't what I wanted, so I felt even more self conscious as I stepped up to serve. The match was to be played over one set. First to win six games would be the school champion of 1985. The match went like this:

Game 1, lost.
Game 2, lost.
Game 3, lost.
Game 4, lost.
Game 5, lost!

As I write this book, 35 years on, I recall the moment as clear as if it was yesterday. I couldn't feel any more battered, embarrassed and deflated. At that moment something clicked inside me. I had reached what I now call my 'bugger it' point. Was I going down with a six to nil result? Maybe, but for goodness sake put a fight up Fernley. For goodness sake, I knew I was better than this. The score wasn't reflecting that the other guy was playing amazingly well, I mean he was playing okay, but I was playing terribly. I hadn't lost my ability to play tennis overnight had I? I hadn't suddenly lost my ability to physically get around the court? What had happened was that I had allowed my mindset to destroy my opportunity to be the best I could be.

I had no idea what was going on in my head back then but I do now. At that point something in my head clicked. Take one shot at a time Fernley. Just play each shot as it comes. That is it. Open the shoulder, let the racket flow and win a point. Shot by shot. Point by point. That is all I had to do to save face, and so after focussing on the ball and breathing (and focusing out the spectators) the scores were as follows; 15 love, 30 love, 50 love, game to me. Wow! Phew!

I went on to win the next six games and take the school championship of 1985. Winning that championship will be something that I will always be proud of. Winning it the way I did will be something I shall never forget. But more than any of that, drawing from these learnings of how the mind can move you from loser to winner was something that has remained with me forever. I have to share this because when we are setting ourselves up for a life changing challenge we have to have the mind in the right place. In my experience it all starts and ends there. Another lesson learned for me that afternoon was the effect of concentrating on one step at a time. No overwhelm, just consistent point by point action that would move me towards where I wanted to be.

The First Calorie-restrictive Diets

Even though in my school years I was very capable at most sports, and won a number of competitions, my weight always knocked my confidence. Kids can be cruel. I'd be ridiculed by other kids at school for being fat. I didn't have a girlfriend until my last few months at school when I eventually hit puberty and started losing the weight. I never really understood why I was overweight. I was active, my parents were slim, and I was good at sport. I grew up in the 70s and 80s where the regular snacking between meals wasn't the norm as it is now. Meal times were quite bland affairs with no particular excess. There was a rule in the house that only two biscuits at a time could be eaten. It was all very simple and minimal. So why was I fat?

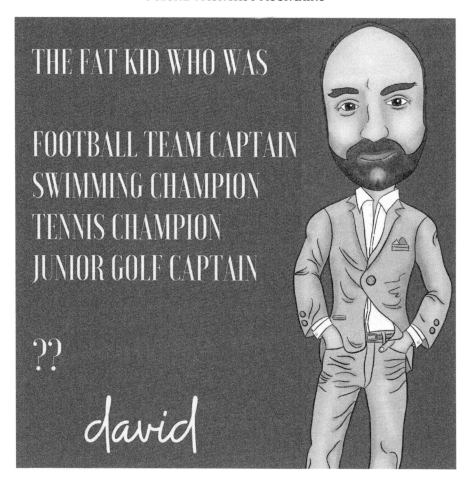

Leaving school and moving to college saw the fat kid slim down to a tall and very thin young man. I was 11.5 stone (161lb, 73kg) and 6'1" at the age of 22. However, with no exercise, a redundancy during a terrible recession, dealing with my parents splitting up, their long and painful divorce, and setting up a business which I was far too young to cope with, I gained 6 stone in weight. I got married to my first wife aged 25 years. I felt fat and bloated at 17.5 stone as I posed for my wedding photographs.

The next few years would see me hover around the 17 stone range as I half-heartedly played with one diet and then the next. However the problem was, I would start on calorific restricted diets so I would end up feeling really hungry and really unhappy. I'd give it a go for two or three weeks and then something would crop up in my life that would take my attention away from my diet and so the diet would stop. What a complete waste of time. This period of my life would see a lot of business stress, a divorce, and a new relationship which would end up as my second marriage, which produced two beautiful kids, Jack and Emma.

Up until this point, despite being naturally good at sport, I had never consistently designed and stuck to a fitness regime. Neither had I ever really designed or stuck to any form of nutritional plan. I loved eating my refined carbs, sweet cakes, fizzy drinks and certainly having a good drink of alcohol.

However, something quite profound happened to me when Jack was a baby and Emma was on her way. I decided that I would start swimming again after years of not being in the pool. I looked around for local pools and found that one of the local health clubs had a 25m pool with a dedicated 'fast lane' for serious swimmers. Looking back I laugh at that thought of being a serious swimmer, because I hadn't swum a single length in years. However, I joined up with the intention of going three or four times a week to try and get some form of fitness back. I'll never forget my first encounter in the fast lane.

Life In The Fast Lane

I turned up with a pair of shorts, I didn't even have a pair of swimming trunks, and I entered the changing rooms. The club had the usual range of members from the super fit no nonsense types through to the heavier, rounder members trying to improve their health, fitness and wellbeing. At 17 stone I was much more the latter. The changing area and showers were a communal affair so I felt extremely conscious of my body.

I entered the pool area and hoped that nobody was in the fast lane. Perhaps I was being a little ambitious to enter that lane, but the right hand lane was full of people just about floating in a forward motion and the central area was people just standing around. I decided that I had to brave the fast lane. Surely it would be okay, after all I had won swimming competitions years ago. So enter the fast I did, and set off on length one. By the time I had reached 25m my heart was pounding and each gasp of air was becoming increasingly forced and stressful. I'll never forget grabbing the blue tiles at the top end of the pool as the realisation of how unfit I was slammed home, hard.

Realising that this swim was going to be a one length at a time affair I gathered myself and pressed on. During my swim a lady got into the fast lane with me. The fast lane was pretty intense as it was only a single lane which was navigated in a clockwise direction. If you committed to a length then you had better be sure to not delay the other swimmers. After the other swimmer got in I had to let her pass me umpteen times as she powered past. I managed 30 single lengths until I finally staggered my way out the pool.

I went home and despite being totally shattered and worried how unfit I had become, I was so pleased that I had been and done it. Despite being conscious of the state that my body had got into, and despite having little confidence, and despite being blown away (and humiliated if I'm honest) by the other swimmer in the fast lane, I was hooked. I had thought that I may return in a couple of days. Bugger that I thought, I'm going back tomorrow!

For the whole of that week I went swimming every day. Within no time I was stringing lengths together and pushing myself further and further, both mentality and physically. I found my ideal time to go to the pool was early in the morning around 6.45am. It was early and all but a couple of serious swimmers were ever in the pool. On occasion, if I was lucky, I'd get into a totally still pool, an experience that was always wonderful.

A couple of weeks went by and I was having a chat with my father on the phone. I mentioned that I had joined the fitness club and that I had started swimming again and that I was loving it. Typically, his reply was that I won't stick to it. Gosh, how to throw a wet blanket onto someone! That was 2002 and as I write this book in 2020 I can still remember how low that thoughtless comment made me feel. Anyone who has struggled with weight will know that transforming your body, mind, health, and wellbeing needs a huge amount of determination, dedication, and support from your nearest and dearest.

Over the next few months I was enjoying swimming and seeing an improvement in my performance. I was keeping up with other swimmers who had previously blasted me away. Some of them I was even overtaking. This felt fantastic. My body had started to change shape and I was not losing weight, I was losing weight fast. I put this weight loss, and body change, down to the swimming alone because I hadn't consciously gone on a diet, but was it really just the swimming? Was this change a result of burning off more energy than I was taking in through the calories in and calories out concept?

Unintentional Intermittent Fasting

My daily routine now was to get up early and go straight to the pool. That meant that I would be out of the club by around 8.15am and off to work during the weekdays and back home at weekends. After a swim I was never really hungry so I would drink some water first and then drink coffee for the rest of the morning. Still being conscious of my extra weight I had started to enjoy the feeling of emptiness, as this made my mid-section feel smaller. I continued enjoying that empty, smaller feeling as the day went on. I felt alive, so with no idea of what was happening to my body as a result of this unintentional daily fast I wouldn't eat anything until at least lunchtime. I'd then eat my usual meal in the evening and perhaps a light snack before bedtime.

As the weight dropped off me, my strength and stamina increased. I was feeling fantastic. I was loving being one of the best swimmers in the club and I have to say that I was starting to look great. My shape was changing into a typical swimmer's physique with wide shoulders tapering down into slim hips. My weight had now dropped to 12 stone 7lbs. I was swimming six days a week, doing weights, running, climbing hills, and eating well. I was happy.

My head was in the place of absolute clarity. I had to exercise everyday, otherwise as my father had so unkindly predicted, I would give all this up as just another temporary fad. So that is what I did. I proved him wrong. My job at the time was Regional Manager for a sports surfacing company. We designed and built synthetic football pitches, hockey pitches, running tracks, and multi-use play areas for school, colleges, universities, and clubs all over the UK. Being an active sportsman was important to me and my job. Having the confidence to meet with premiership football clubs and famous managers needed a level of confidence that was lacking in my fatter days. I would travel a lot and my job was demanding. Despite that, I would make maximum effort to get some form of exercise session in every day. If I had to miss a day then I would feel guilty. That guilt, and the fear of failure, kept me going.

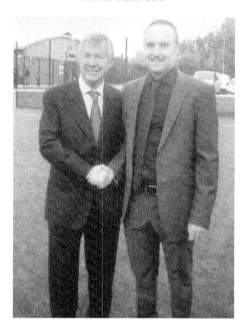

With Sir Alex Ferguson in April 2010. This was the launch of the multi-million pound sports facility at Partington Sports Village, which is part of Broad Oak High School, Trafford.

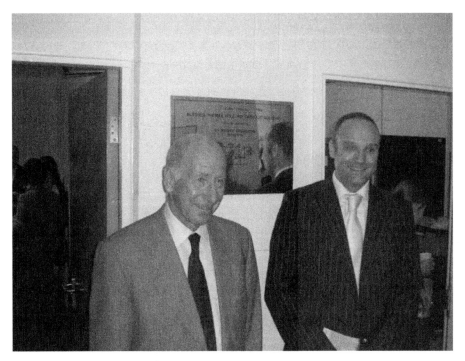

With Sir Bobby Charlton in April 2007 at Blessed Thomas Holford Catholic College, Altrincham, for the opening of a new synthetic sports pitch.

My First Big Challenge

During my time swimming I got to know a regular who was simply a machine in the pool. He was super fit. We matched each other length for length over long distances. He asked me if I wanted to swim the length of Lake Windermere with him and would I consider doing the English Channel. Hell yes, was my answer. However a problem arose, I had started to experience an aching in my right shoulder which led to stiffness and pain. I had also noticed that when playing ball with the kids, or throwing a ball for the dogs, my shoulder hurt and I was losing power. This stiffness gradually got worse to a point whereby I was forced to see a specialist sports injury consultant who gave me the most painful injection deep into my shoulder. Six months of physiotherapy followed, and that unfortunately put a stop to my planned challenges.

However disappointing my shoulder problem was, I kept swimming and training, and I just changed my sessions to suit. I got pretty good at doing the front crawl one armed. It is important to mention that during this time, despite my injury, my confidence was still soaring. I was able to buy whatever clothes I wanted and I felt great in them. I even started wearing the slimline type shirts and tops just because I could. It was the first time in my life that I could wear such clothes and gosh, was I going to make the most of it!

I was at a barbecue one evening, whilst visiting my wife's family in Canada, when an older guy, who would have been in his late 60s and had suffered a lot of ill health, said something very memorable to me. We were talking about health and fitness and he said, 'Lad, when you get to my age you will REALLY appreciate the efforts you are putting in now. Always keep your body as young as possible'.

Gosh, yes, to this day I recall that conversation as clear as day.

The Black Dog

2010 arrived and so did my 40th birthday. Things weren't going right in my marriage and after a painful few years, my wife and I decided to separate. Also in that same year the company that I worked for went into administration as a casualty of the recession. This job was more than just a job to me. I loved what I did and I had some great friends there too. I had grown and developed massively over that period and this loss would hit me hard. I'd noticed a change in my mood over a period of time which developed into something much deeper. Over the next few months I was diagnosed with anxiety and depression and prescribed anti-depressant tablets. I wasn't in a good place.

This period on my life was extremely difficult. Depression is awful. It is the most dreadful of conditions. I remember afternoons where I would sleep to escape my feelings only to awaken to the sinking feeling of dread. Keeping fit was a help to me during this time, but I was finding the motivation to keep going increasingly difficult.

I found a new job, still within the sports industry, but the head office was in Paris which meant a huge amount of travel throughout not only the UK but Europe too. This completely disrupted my training schedule. Most evenings were spent drinking and eating out and my diet soon became compromised.

It was during this time that I met Amanda. This was the most positive news and I can't thank her enough for the help and support she gave me during those times. However, Amanda lived an hour away across the Pennines and as we developed our relationship, and spent more time together, I stopped swimming. Gradually my trips to the pool lessened. I remember one particular day sitting in the steam room after a swim, a swim that I had struggled with, noticing the belly that was starting to bulge over my swimming trunks. Very quickly the slow-down in routine, the stresses of that period, and the increased drinking and eating out was starting to show.

My health and fitness routine went downhill very quickly from that point. I was unaware then of the effects that the stress hormone cortisol has on fat storage. Stopping the exercise, and too many meals out with wines and beer were showing in my body very quickly. During this period I also found myself in a bitter divorce and an even bitter fight to keep seeing my kids. A fight which was totally unnecessary, and fuelled by jealousy and hatred. My savings were being drained very quickly on solicitors and barristers so the last thing I cared about was my health and fitness.

The following ten years has been a period of consistent fat gain with a number of side effects manifesting themselves. During this ten year period I would find myself getting into a habit of drinking alcohol on a daily basis. In our home I am the cook. I enjoy cooking, and I certainly enjoy cooking with a drink or two whilst playing my favourite music in the background. This was 'my time' during the day. The stresses of the business day had been dealt with, and now was the time to crack open a bottle of lager and chill out. The problem was that a couple of drinks led to three, four, and more. Beer changed to wine, and wine changed to spirits. The regular drinking became a daily regime and at weekends I might even have a couple of beers at lunchtime. My family was starting to get worried and I couldn't blame them.

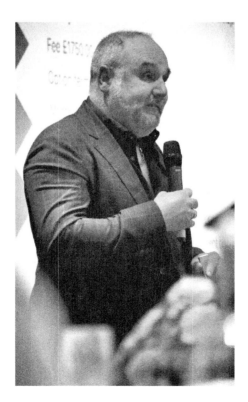

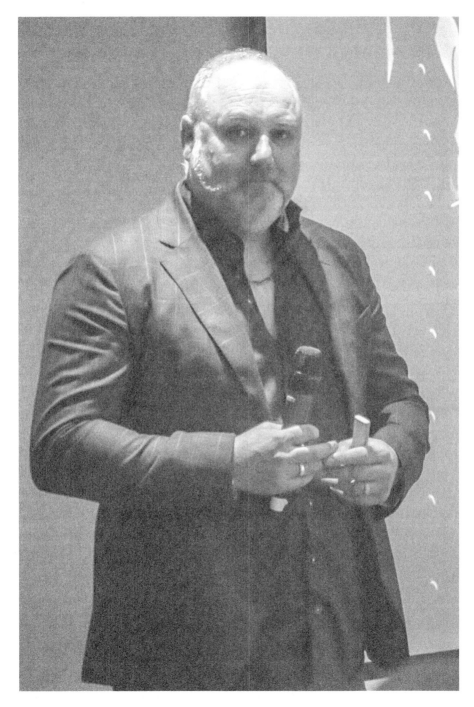

Swimming in d'Nile

Around eight years ago I started to suffer with indigestion and heartburn which is pretty awful. I found some great tablets which I could buy over the counter and so the problem was solved. At least that is what I told myself. These tablets would now be a daily medication. If I didn't take one then the burning and the acid would be awful. Amanda suggested that I may have an ulcer and that I should have this checked out. I ignored her. I didn't want a camera pushing down my throat, but whilst I ignored Amanda I knew that if this continued then there would be a real possibility of contracting cancer. However, that fear didn't focus my mind into sorting myself out.

Another ailment that came from nowhere, and around the time of my new acid problems were callouses on my feet. I'd never had callouses before. I put this down to living in a house with painted hardwood flooring rather than carpet. Over this period we had lived in two farmhouses with a mix of wooden flooring, tiles, and York stone flags. I was convinced that walking around with bare feet was the cause of this painful condition. However, I did start to question that theory when I bought slippers. I'd wear the slippers, use a pumice stone on my feet, keep them moisturised, but still nothing changed. Amanda and the kids walked barefoot on the same floors and their feet were fine. The callouses always cracked into deep slits and these slits were incredibly painful. My feet were that hard my daughter Emma said that they were made of stone.

The last in the trio of ailments was the snoring. For years my long suffering bed sharer has had to sleep with ear plugs. The snoring could get so bad that I would wake up with a sore and swollen throat. I'll mention sleep in more detail later on in the book, but I can tell you now that I'd never had a full night's sleep. I'd wake up through sleep apnea, reflux, or snoring. The reflux would have me waking in a panic, unable to breathe, struggling with fear and desperation until I could start to breathe again. Perhaps more damaging was falling asleep every night on the sofa as we settled down to watch something good on TV. I simply couldn't help it. I literally couldn't keep my eyes open. This wasn't fair on Amanda and the kids. This sleeping caused many a ruined evening but I just couldn't help it.

It was clear that my weight and poor health was causing problems. If this was what was happening on the outside of my body, goodness knows what was happening on the inside. What about the full physiological and psychological effects of weight gain and poor health?

Have you ever got to the point of not wanting to take your top off in summer for fear of looking bad? Even worse have you ever got to the point of wanting to hide your body from the person that you are in love with? As a speaker I've never watched a video of myself presenting. You may ask why? It's because I couldn't stand to look at my fat body and my fat face on film. I hated it. Over the past ten years all of that confidence I enjoyed in the previous slim and fit years disappeared. I hated the way I looked and I felt it.

There was no doubt that in order to make the huge life changes that I had to make, I would need to plan this transformation out. I would need to formulate a plan which was liveable, sustainable, and get me the results I desperately needed. This plan would take into account my current position and get me from where I was, to where I wanted to be. I've named this plan The Personal Purpose Plan™.

CHAPTER 2

The Personal Purpose Plan™

T his chapter explores where my position was in terms of health, fitness, and nutrition. The Personal Purpose Plan™ looks at demands in terms of available time and challenges effecting lifestyle. When I started my transformation I explored my own challenges and set the goal and plan in terms of my desired weight, fitness, and lifestyle.

Facing Up To Lockdown

So this brings me to March 2020, Covid-19, and Lockdown. As it was for many people, Covid-19 was severely damaging our business and it was looking like Amanda and I were going to be among the directors and small businesses that the Government didn't look after with grants and giveaways. We couldn't hold events and people were scared of spending money. This was getting very serious, very quickly, and I was getting very worried.

As Lockdown was looking inevitable Amanda and I went out to stock up on food for a family of four. No, we didn't panic buy (honest!) but we bought a week's worth of shopping on the Tuesday evening. As we got back to the farm and pulled the car up, I grabbed the chain from the back of the car that locks the main gate and for some reason took a photo of it. It was at that point I realised that we were completely out of control in this whole horrible situation. I went back to the house, poured myself a large gin and tonic, and sat on my own thinking and asking myself the following questions. What could we do? Could we make the most of these times? How long would this Lockdown thing be? How could I use this time? What could I do in this time to better our lives? I came up with a few answers, but one answer would be the clearest and most important by far. I would get back to a great level of health and fitness.

Yes, this felt right. Over the past ten years I'd had umpteen false starts where I'd start rowing for a couple of weeks and then I'd give up. I'd let business get in the way, or I'd get a cold and stop, or I'd just get fed up and give in. This time it *had* to be different. I wasn't feeling particularly well and I knew that all this forthcoming time on my hands had to be the best opportunity I had to work on the greatest asset I had - my body. Rather than let this new virus be a negative in my life, I was going to take advantage of another huge asset, time, and sort myself out.

Lockdown had presented me with an opportunity. If I was going to replicate the results of 2002-2010 I would need to set a goal and then set out how I would achieve that goal.

Strategy and Accountability

Most endeavours in life need some form of strategy. I knew that to lose at least five stone in weight over five months, and get fit, strong, and healthy at the same time would take some form of plan. If I didn't get the strategy right then I would very likely fail, give up, and stay fat.

Having surgery wasn't an option for me. Whilst I can appreciate this may work for some, there was no way that I was putting myself through that. I've witnessed friends pick at a cold meal for ninety minutes, unable to eat properly, because of a gastric band. No, this wasn't for me. I knew from my previous life that there were many interdependent elements to losing fat and getting fit and I knew that in my middle age this was never more important.

As a form of accountability I posted a photograph of myself with Sir Alex Ferguson at one of our football pitch openings on my Facebook profile. Even if I say so myself, it's a great photo of me and Alex! But incredibly, nobody on Facebook thought it was me. I was unrecognisable. At the time that photograph was taken I was around 14 stone and I was super fit. Wouldn't it be fantastic if I could get back to that weight. Would this be possible though at the age of 50?

Whilst nobody had any idea how long Lockdown would be in place, I guessed that our events business and normal work routine wouldn't return until well after the summer. This would mean that I had five months until the end of August to transform my body back to what it was. I weighed myself. I was 19 stone 2lb (269lb, 121kg). This would mean a drop in weight of 5 stone in 5 months. If I could pull this off then it would be a massive success.

There would have to be a number of huge changes to put into place and these changes would have to be phased in. I knew me well enough and I knew that unless I put into place a strategy and a programme, then the chances of pulling this off would be little to none with me giving up again over the next week or two. This time had to, and would, be different.

Operation Lockdown

Stage 1(a)

I would need to exercise every day and that exercise would have to be varied and carefully considered. I was extremely unfit and my body was stiff. Running would stress my joints and the high pulse and blood pressure rates worried me. Exercise using my own body weight would be difficult as I had an obesely heavy body and very poor strength. I would need to concentrate on aerobic exercise whilst gradually introducing more resistance training. I had the time so why not get up and get out in the morning and also get on the rowing machine and weights in the late afternoon/early evening? Yes, I could do that.

Stage 1(b)

The elimination of snacks, late night cheese and biscuits, cake, crisps, sugar, take outs, fizzy sugary and sweetened drinks, and processed supermarket ready meals.

Stage 1(c)

I would study nutrition and fitness. I wasn't 32 years old this time. I was three months off the big 5-0 with a very different body than that of 18 years ago. I wanted to make sure, as sure as I could be, that my diet was going to be sustainable for me and that I would get maximum benefit. Lockdown had presented me with time to study, time that could be easily designed around my new routine. Total flexibility.

Stage 2(a)

I would start designing my meal plan. Lean meats, an increase in fish consumption, reducing and being selective on the carbohydrates. Proteins, and fats would be the basis of my meals. I'd introduce more fibre and take on more fruit and vegetables.

Stage 2(b)

Try and take in at least a gallon of fresh spring water every day. We live on a farm that is supplied by a bore hole, meaning that we have fresh spring water coming out of our taps. The water is UV treated so we don't have the taste of other people's kidneys along with the added chemicals in our water, you know...the tastes that the water companies say we can't taste.

Drinking water is an absolute must. Whilst the health benefits of drinking water are huge, for hydration and clarity, water also helps with appetite and hunger pangs. I knew that should I ever feel hungry then an ice cold glass of water took that edge off. I would also drink a glass of water as soon as I got up in the morning. For many years the first job of the day would be to put the coffee machine on and enjoy at least six cups of white, sugared coffee. How crazy! After a night's sleep we are dehydrated. We need water to hydrate ourselves so that at least our poor brain can work properly.

Another benefit I noticed, was that my daily headaches disappeared. It became habit to pop a paracetamol or two almost every day. I have to apologise to Amanda who kept telling me that it was the water I took with the headache tablets that cured the headache, rather than the tablets themselves. Don't tell her, for goodness sake, but she was right! I rarely have a headache these days.

(I'm editing your book, I'll make you apologise to my face later! ~Amanda)

Rather than just drinking plain water in the morning, I'd also enjoy a pint of fresh lemon water. As well as increasing hydration, a glass of warm water with freshly squeezed lemon, is a great source of vitamin C. Lemon water also supports weight loss, improves skin quality, aids digestion, freshens breath, and helps prevent kidney stones. It would be a no-brainer to enjoy a glass of fresh lemon water surely. Green tea, ginger tea, and lemon tea would replace the usual fizzy sugary and sweetened drinks. Each of these teas has numerous health benefits and are a hugely beneficial replacement to costly sweet drinks with no nutritional value whatsoever.

Stage 3

The elimination of alcohol. Not that I would be counting calories, but to give you an idea of where I was, I was consuming in excess of 5000 calories per week through alcoholic drinks. Putting aside for one moment the huge health risks of drinking that much, I would never be able to out-train that level of alcohol. I knew that unless I cut the booze I could train as hard as I wanted, stress my body, get totally fed up, but see nothing change. What was the point in doing a fitness session to burn up to 800 calories and then go and put them all back in later that same evening? I would need to cut the alcohol totally until I had reached my target and then only resume alcohol, should I want to, in moderation.

Stage 4

Intermittent fasting. The control of insulin levels in the body is crucial to the effects of fat loss. I shall go further into this later in the book, but the calories in/calories out beliefs of the past few decades have been proven to be an absolute nonsense with failure and disappointing results for most people. Keeping the insulin hormone down is crucial as is the control of the stress hormone cortisol. Fasting is essential to the control of insulin levels and so I would need to integrate this into my regime.

Stage 5

Sleep and relax. As briefly mentioned above, stress causes fat storage. Cortisol is the stress hormone. Cortisol is affected by stress caused by anxiety and too much anaerobic exercise. After years of piling weight on during the last stressful decade, it would be important to work on reducing my stress levels as well as being very careful with the intensity of exercise I would undertake. Sleep would also be extremely important. I would need to get a good night's sleep every night which seemed an impossibility considering the reflux, and sleep apnea that I had suffered for years.

Stage 6

The slow increase in exercise as my fitness and stamina levels also slowly increase. My concentration needed to be on consistent aerobic exercise which would burn energy and, in co-ordination with fasting, would burn that stubborn visceral fat as effectively as possible. Visceral fat is the dangerous yellow fat that builds up around your organs.

Resistance training would also be very important. As I lose fat I would need to transition to more resistance and muscle building training. It's a common misunderstanding that doing intensive core exercises will 'burn fat' and produce that much desired six pack. It won't. You may build muscle sure, but it will just be covered in fat. You need to burn the fat first. There is a saying that you won't find your abs in the gym, you'll find them in the kitchen. Reduce your body fat through good food, and only then will you find your abs.

So that was the target and that was the masterplan. Now I had to decide what would help me keep this regime up?

Accountability Counts In Large Amounts

Having been a property mentor for a number of years, I had witnessed the power of accountability in our clients' success. Accountability is an incredibly important motivator in any training programme. It was clear to me that to achieve these goals I would need to make myself accountable to someone. The first obvious choice was Amanda, Jack, and Emma. However, they had seen umpteen false starts before so why would they take this attempt seriously this time? So who else could I make myself accountable too?

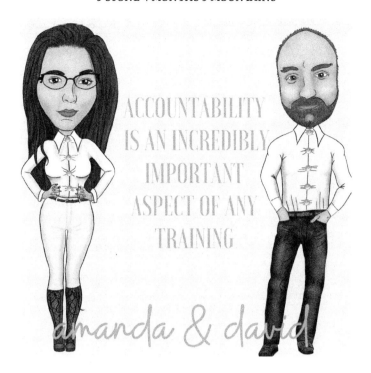

Well, there were my friends on Facebook. Almost 5000 of them. If I posted my goal then I would have publicly made a statement, so that is what I did. I posted my intention on 25 March 2020 and I received 116 wonderful messages of support. I posted a few days later on the same subject and received 134 messages of support. Another accountability post received 161 amazing comments. How could I not be accountable now to these well-wishers? I'd put myself out there and everyone knew, so hiding or making excuses would be a lot harder to bear. At the same time I was receiving lots of personal messages of support from friends informing me that my efforts has inspired them to do the same thing. This was truly wonderful.

My accountability wouldn't stop there. What if I committed to do some sort of fitness test and do it for charity? Something, that in March 2020 I would have zero chance of pulling off? I had always wanted to climb a mountain but never had. I had heard about the National Three Peaks Challenge and how it had to be completed within 24 hours.

The National Three Peaks Challenge consists of climbing the three highest mountains of Scotland, England, and Wales. The total walking distance is 23 miles (37km) and the total ascent is 3064 metres (10,052ft). Including the driving, the challenge is to complete this within 24 hours. I spoke to Peter, and with Amanda along to do the driving, we decided to do it. As this challenge involves climbing mountains in the middle of the night, we would need to do this as close to mid-summer as possible. Taking Lockdown into account and hoping we could, we decided to start the challenge on 27 July 2020. This would give me just three months to train. We chose the homeless charity Crisis and I set up a Just Giving page. There was a lot to do. There was no way that I'd be wanting to drag 19 stone up and down three mountains. I'd have to hit this weight loss and training hard.

Another crucial aspect to achieving my goals would be consistency. Something positive in my fitness and nutrition regime had to happen every single day without fail and it had to be sustainable. By setting out the plan in small bitesize steps I wouldn't put myself into shock, overwhelm and overload. By slightly increasing every stage of the plan, every day, I would create regular psychological wins. I knew from my early swimming days that this would work.

The slight increases and changes that I would be constantly making would have the effect of gradual improvement without the shock to the system that causes the early failures for so many New Year resolutions.

Time Is Relative

My relationship with time would be crucial to succeeding and I encourage you to consider your relationship with time very carefully too. In my swimming days I spoke with so many friends and work colleagues who would always say that they could never find the time to swim, go to the gym, or even have enough time to put on a pair of running shoes and go out for a short run.

I've also heard friends and colleagues talk about not having enough time in the morning to prepare themselves something healthy for lunch. They also did not have time to cook a healthy whole food meal in the evening. They only had time to grab a drive thru or ping a supermarket ready meal in the microwave. If I'm honest, I've said exactly the same during the bad times. It's crap!

This isn't because you, or they, or I, don't have the time. It is because we use lack of time as an excuse because we don't really want to put the time in to look after our health. Let's for one moment consider intermittent fasting. What time do we need to fast? None! In fact fasting saves us time. We don't have to do anything. No shopping, no food preparation, no cooking, no eating, no clearing up, and then we don't feel sluggish and tired after eating. I'll be going through intermittent fasting in more detail later in the book.

- How long does it take to prepare a glass of lemon water in the morning? No more than 20 seconds. Set your alarm clock one minute earlier.

- How long does it take to make a garlic mushroom omelette garnished with fresh parsley? Around 10 minutes if you have to crush the clove yourself.

- How long does it take to put a piece of salmon in the oven, boil some new potatoes, put a couple of vegetables in a pan, and then serve? 25 minutes maximum!

We have 24 hours in a day. If we take out one hour to exercise that leaves us with 23 hours. Take off 7 hours to sleep and that leaves us with 16 hours. Let's take 11 hours to commute and work and that leaves us with 5 hours of family time. Can't you really find an hour to work on yourself, for you and your family? I'll discuss time and time management in more detail later.

I knew that I had to carefully plan my time. I would design my regime to utilise those 24 hours in the day to gain fitness and lose weight.

There Is No Fun In Failure and No Failure in Fun

Having fun with this would also be crucial to the success of my goals in not only achieving my results, but to ensure continuity into the future. There is absolutely nothing appealing in having a fitness schedule if you hate the diet and hate the exercise. There is only one outcome and that is to stop, to stop the misery! I knew that to embrace my plan and make it succeed I would need to enjoy what I'm eating and I would need to look forward to my daily exercise. During my prior eight years of fitness I had thoroughly enjoyed swimming, running, and punchbag work. I enjoyed each sport and as it was varied, nothing ever got stale.

This time though I couldn't swim due to Lockdown, neither could I join a gym for the same reason. I also didn't have my punchbag anymore. So rather than focus on what I didn't have, I focussed on what I did have. I have some great countryside to train in. I had a bike to have fun on. I could grab the kids and go for a hike, and then mix that up with our rowing machine and use what weights I had, if I could find them in the back of the garage. I could vary my exercise and have fun at the same time.

The diet wasn't going to a diet in the traditional sense. Rather than deprivation and denial I just switched to eating the healthy foods that I enjoyed whilst gradually replacing and dropping the unhealthy foods. My primary goal was to ensure that I enjoyed every meal.

- I love roast salmon in lemon and pepper, so I ate it.
- I love steak, so I ate it.
- I love Thai green and Thai red curry, so I ate plenty.
- I love king prawns, so I ate them.
- I love fresh tuna steaks, so I ate them.
- I love mussels, scallops, and squid, so I ate them.
- I love cashew nuts, so I added them to some meals.
- I love eggs. We have chickens so they are the freshest most free range eggs we knew, and I ate them.

Scrapping pizza, crisps, milk chocolate, biscuits, fizzy drinks, chips and pies was no bother whatsoever. I knew that I wouldn't miss them because I was going to enjoy better quality food. Plus the shelves in the shops had been cleared by food hoarders so that made it a lot easier because I couldn't be tempted even if I wanted to be!

Studying My Way To Success

I read, studied, and learned as much as I could so that I could maximise the effort and time I was investing so that everything I did, or didn't do, was pushing towards the goal.

- I read books on nutrition. I signed up for and passed diploma courses on nutrition. I watched umpteen nutrition related documentaries on Netflix and listened to even more podcasts on the subject.

- I also learned how counting calories was not going to help me sustain a weight that I could maintain into the future. At almost 50 years old I had to be smarter than I was 18 years ago when my body was a very different body to what it is now.

- I knew that no amount of training would compensate for consuming a huge amounts of calories through a bad diet with alcohol. An example of this was the 5000 plus calories a week that I was drinking because of my alcohol habit. Purely on a calorie in and calorie out basis (which I don't subscribe to as I shall explain later in the book), I would need to train hard for five days, burning 1000 per day, just to burn the G&Ts off. How crazy!

· I now knew that eating and snacking at the wrong times would keep my insulin levels up and stop my body from burning stubborn fat stores, especially the dangerous visceral fat around my organs.

· I knew now that drinking the wrong fluids would damage the result that I was aiming for. Sugary drinks would spike the insulin levels. Artificially sweetened drinks have exactly the same effects! Whilst sweeteners have no calories, they still spike those insulin levels which means that no amount of exercise will burn those fat reserves.

· I learned that eating at the right times would be crucial. My intention was to introduce fasting which would hugely help insulin reduction and the body's ability to burn fat.

· I learned that exercising a 50 year old body was very different than exercising a 30 years old body. I knew that doing the wrong type of exercise would damage my results in the earlier stages of fat loss. Cortisol is the stress hormone which encourages the body to store fat. If I adopted the old 'no pain no gain' type of training then I'd only raise my cortisol levels and reduce the effectiveness of fat burning exercise. I'd probably also stop altogether because I hated that high intensity type of exercise.

· I discovered that simple techniques such as training at the correct times would also be crucial. Training whilst in a fasted state produces growth hormones which is perfect when building and conditioning muscle. Training whilst in a fasted state would also accelerate the body's ability to burn fat far quicker than when training in a non-fasted state.

- I also learned that sleeping would be extremely important. The body needs to rest and repair. I've studied so many people who have all recognised the difference in not only performance, but weight gain, when not taking the correct amount of sleep.

Finally, I would hold dear people of a similar mind who had, or was, engaging in the same regime that I was to undertake. Having friends who totally understand what you are trying to achieve, and will support you, is crucial in anything that is worth doing in life.

In this book I am going to break down the remaining main elements of what has got me to achieve, and surpass, my goals.

The plan had now been set. Now the mindset had been switched into place. I told myself that I had to achieve my goals and nothing would stop me from regaining my health. This was happening! I take pleasure in introducing The Motivated Mindset Matrix™.

CHAPTER 3

The Motivated Mindset Matrix™

W hat has made us get to where we are now? What will get us where we want to be? What will keep us in this brilliant new state for the long term? Mindset is critical and if we are to transform for the better then we need put ourselves in an absolute state of certainty. There must be no doubt in our goals.

When the decision was made to get myself fit again, Amanda didn't take my undertaking very seriously. In fact she didn't have any faith in me at all. I could recognise her doubt through her raised eyebrow whenever I mentioned doing exercise and losing weight again. I can't really blame her, I had promised the same promise umpteen times over the past few years, but had failed each and every time. I didn't make a fuss about this, I just posted my commitment on social media, and I decided that finally this had to happen. Deep down I knew, at the age of 49, that unless I got to grips with my health then at some point something chronic would catch up with me.

Taking That First Step

I recall going to bed one evening, only a few months ago, lying on my bed and feeling dreadful. I had drunk alcohol that night, eaten a take-out pizza, and fallen asleep again on the sofa, which never went down well with my family. As I lay there feeling terrible I came to the realisation that if I kept going the way I was going then my life expectancy would be significantly short-ened. Something would get me; heart disease, cancer, diabetes, a heart attack? Then that would be that. *Dead!*

Laying there that night, feeling bad, was reason enough to finally get my head in the right place to make a change; but why only concentrate on the negative aspects of health and fitness, and only motivate myself through fear? Why not also concen-trate on all of the fantastic aspects of being slimmer, fitter, and healthier? Being able to enjoy climbing mountains with friends, being able to actually find clothes that fit me, feeling confident again, being able to run, swim, cycle properly again. Feeling a sense of pride when I look at a photo, rather than scrapping most of them because they are unflattering, and too honest for me to bear.

Recognising what had worked for me in the past had taught me a lot. Observing people who had made huge changes in their lives (as well as the people who never seemed to successfully make the changes they desire) had also taught me a lot. I learned that achieving any major change in life required momentum. I had to start and I had to start now. So many people, including my-self, talk about doing something but then never follow through. They never take that first step. Talking about doing something is so easy, too easy, and you can kid yourself for a looooong time. But I would take that first step and I'd anchor into a state that would inspire me to succeed.

Motivation Has To Come From Deep Within

I dug out an old photograph of when I was six stone lighter and super fit. It was a photograph of me and my son Jack in Las Vegas after I had just completed a two mile swim. I remember that time like it was yesterday and I remember how great I felt. I imagined myself at that peak state by remembering how great

I felt then and how confident I was then. I could return to that body over the next few months. If I could concentrate and focus on how great I felt then, then that should give me the momentum to change.

The next thing I did was to get passionate about this change. I knew how great I could feel, if I got my old body back. That is all well and good and positive and happy, but I also got passionate about how bad I felt now. I looked at myself in the mirror. I really looked at myself with honesty in the mirror, without skimming over the bad bits. I looked at the videos of me speaking on stage, and I even took screenshots of the really unflattering angles. I went and dug out the bottles of gin in the recycling bin and lined them up. I admitted to myself how much I was was drinking.

I drafted a post to put onto Facebook and I chose my words very carefully. I didn't use soft words like overweight, or heavy, I used the word fat. I would get passionate about being fat because I knew that by jolting myself into action, I would have a greater chance of success. I then considered what would life be for Amanda, Jack, and Emma if I became ill. Even worse, what if I became ill and died. How could I not get myself healthy again for them? I found my emotions. These emotions would push me forward to make the life changing decisions I had to make.

This is where the decision to start had now become real. I was acting upon that decision. Perhaps the biggest action I could have possibly taken was to post this acknowledgement on social media with before and after photographs. One with fit me from years ago, next to fat me speaking on stage. It took some courage to post on Facebook but I did it. I held myself accountable not only my family, my personal friends, my clients, my mentees, but people whom I had never met and never spoken to. This was huge for me. As the messages of goodwill came in, and the likes, one after another, I knew this was it. It was time to get fit and healthy again.

FOOD HAD BECOME A FRIEND, A SOCIAL PASTIME, SOMETHING TO ALLEVIATE BOREDOM, A COMFORT IN TIMES OF NEGATIVITY, AND A TREAT

david

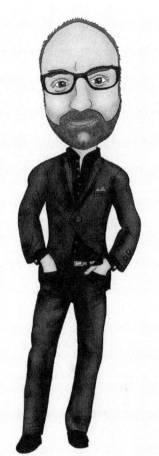

Now I had my passion; both the positive and the negative passion, I had to decide what I was to do with that passion. I had to start and follow through with massive action on the passion that I was feeling. Today I would start. Today I would start with a change in diet and I would put my walking boots on and walk. This is where the decision to start had now become real. I was acting upon that decision. Perhaps the biggest action I could have possibly taken was to post in social media with before and after photographs. One with me fit, next to one with me fat. It took some courage to post on Facebook but I did. I held myself accountable not only my family, my personal friends, my clients, my mentees, but people whom I had never met and never spoken to. This was huge for me. As the messages of goodwill came in, one after another, after another, and so on, I knew this was it. It was time to get fit and healthy again.

Dealing With The Everyday Obstacles

I knew that as I progressed and pushed through the first stages of the journey, I would encounter obstacles that could throw me off the plan. There would be times when I looked in the mirror and my mind would tell me that I wasn't making good enough progress. There would be times when the scales wouldn't move as I would expect them to. There would be times when the body was saying no and I would need to step back to let the body recover.

These obstacles would be expected and I needed to embrace them and accept them because they would be real to me. I would recognise them for what they were and push on, but there may be a need to change my strategy over the next few months. A 19 stone plus unhealthy man is a very different to a 13 stone super fit athlete. I would need to keep monitoring my progress and make the changes as required. There is nothing more constant than change. Having my ultimate focus on the goal I had set would mean that if the results weren't working then I would need to change. If that didn't work then I would change again, and I would keep changing until my goal was reached.

I knew that emotion would play a huge part in this. I put myself in the mindset that I had to succeed. If I missed an exercise session then I would feel guilty. If I snacked on rubbish food then I would feel guilty. If I wasn't achieving my results then I would feel enough frustration to change and push smarter and harder. At the same time the feelings of appreciation and support from the people that I loved was priceless. The feelings of seeing the kilos drop off me and throwing away clothes that were now far too big for me was exhilarating.

All of this was great, and would get me to where I wanted to get to, but what about the dreaded thing that had destroyed my health and fitness in the past and made me unrecognisable to the man I was? Stress!

Stress During Lockdown

The world was experiencing something new and unprecedented. Covid-19 had gone from just something on the news in some area in China to a killer virus that was closing down businesses and lifestyles right here on our doorstep. We were entering Lockdown, a term that we would all get very used to using, but nobody really understood what that meant.

Pubs were closing. Cafes, shops, meeting places, weddings, churches, offices, factories, health clubs, swimming pools, everything was closing and being cancelled! More immediately worrying for us was that our education business was not able to hold events anymore. If we could not hold training events, how could we generate income? Yes we could move online but doing that wasn't an overnight solution and even with online courses, was anyone buying? People were in fear of losing their businesses, income, jobs, and homes, so would they be spending on education? We didn't have a clue. Nobody did.

Other immediate worries were how the income streams from our properties were going to be affected. Were our tenants going to be able to keep paying their rent? Would mortgage companies keep wanting their monthly fees along with council tax payments, insurances, and utilities? Was this suspension on everything we knew going to mean recession or even economic depression? What would happen to house prices? Would they plunge which could mean we would find ourselves in huge negative equity again? The fears were real and this nightmare was escalating daily as the implications and ramifications started to sink in.

I knew that stress had destroyed my health over the last ten years through constant worrying. I knew now that unless I dealt with these worries the best I could, and quickly, that my health mission would shudder to a halt or maybe not even get started at all. If I allowed these fears to grow and dominate my headspace I'd no doubt return to helpless inactivity, bad food, and the booze.

When Stress and Worry Ruled

In the past I'd let worrying and negative thoughts throw my attention from doing exercise sessions, eating the right things, and having fun. I let these thoughts push me towards comfort foods and comfort eating and of course to drown my sorrows in a bottle of wine, a few beers, or something harder. I'd allow this negativity to completely demotivate me and prevent me getting out and doing fitness sessions. Then as the weight started to creep on, I lost more motivation. The stress was allowed to dominate my head, and everything went downhill very fast. I wasn't going to allow this to happen again.

Worries are simply thoughts in your head which should be dealt with quickly, one way or another. When I look back on my life, most of the worries that dominated my thinking never materialised into actual real life issues that could hurt us. Worries that did actually materialise, always got dealt with when they happened. I look back and ask myself why I let worries get me down so much. I'm still here. I live with my family whom I love dearly. I live in a beautiful house. I have cash in the bank and I retain income-producing assets dating back to the 1990s from when I was a young man. Not one of the crazy thoughts that caused me anxiety and depression had actually ruined anything in my life.

We can pretty much deal with anything that comes our way, so why worry about stuff that hasn't happened? Why let nothing-much-at-all cause so much anxiety? Surely the only time to pay any attention to something negative is when we actually have to deal with the issue? Recognise that there is an issue, if it even exists, and deal with it at the appropriate time. If the issue can't be dealt with now, then put it into a box, label it, shelve it and deal with it as soon as you can.

A practice that I have developed recently is to write down any worrying niggles on paper and then stop worrying about them until I have to, or until I have time to address them. Worries that are allowed to float around your head grow and grow like ever inflating balloons of doom and you end up losing all perspective. Worries get bigger and bigger so write them down and see how small (or daft) they really are.

A recent example I can give you is a dispute that I have with someone over a business matter. I received a ridiculous email over the weekend which initially really got under my skin as I knew it was totally wrong. For a number of reasons this matter doesn't need dealing with yet but it was on my mind all afternoon. I was due to do my afternoon exercise session, and wham, here we go again, I didn't want to do any exercise. I wanted to brood on this ridiculous situation instead, just like I did in the old days.

I took a deep breath and reminded myself that I had a goal, that I had a strategy to achieve my goal, and that I had made myself accountable on social media. I simply wrote a quick draft email reply and filed it. There, I had got all of the negativity out of my head and into the email where it belonged. I then exercised as planned feeling so much better about the matter and myself. The session was good, and I was pleased that I had done it, and then I was able to enjoy the rest of the evening knowing that I had done the right thing. I ended up deleting that email because it wasn't even worth replying to in the end.

A Stressful Business

If you are reading this and you have a stressful business, or have a demanding job that has affected your health then the chances are you will resonate with at least some of this.

It was during a particularly busy period in the serviced accommodation business when I went to see the doctor. I had started to experience my head getting hot, red, with the feelings of pressure in my face. Whilst it's often good to be busy, this period wasn't a particularly good and productive type of busy. We were having issues with the housekeeping which meant that I was forced to go back and run everything on site.

In the cleaning business, finding good reliable staff is a huge issue. I've never met a cleaner who went through school with the ambition of being a cleaner. Neither have I ever heard of a careers advice officer suggesting that someone ought to consider a career in cleaning. Being a cleaner is a job that people don't really aspire to. In other words, the vast majority of people who clean do it because they have little or no choice. This was the case with our team, including our sub-contractors, and it showed. Absent days, late starts, sloppy or missed work, inflating the hours actually worked.

In the hotel and hospitality business guests want a 100% immaculately presented property and many of them want to check in earlier than advertised, but they want to check out later than they should, and then they leave the place as a complete dump before the next guest wants to check in early. This put added pressure on a team who are not particularly motivated from the outset as they are doing a job that they don't particularly want to do. So these were some of the reasons I had to go back and run operations.

At the same time Amanda was having her own struggles with her administrative team. What this meant was a period of stress both at work and at home. Being a married couple in business can be great, but this can very easily lead to the business overwhelming a marriage and the family home. There was simply no escape from the pressures of work during this time.

The doctor checked my blood pressure and advised me to go back regularly to monitor what was going on, but of course, I ignored Amanda and the doctor and buried my head in denial.

24/7, 365, ...Never Ending Stress!

We were running a 24/7, 365 days a year business, and it was intense. I would get up around 6am having not slept properly due to my snoring, reflux, and sleep apnea. I'd pack all of the linens and consumables, drop the kids off at school, and then spend 90 minutes sat in traffic to get to either Manchester, Leeds, or Bradford. I'd pick up a latte en route, probably a super size one, and by the time I'd sugared it (3 sugar sticks!) I'd be taking in around 400 calories right there and then, with just one drink.

Depending on which route I was driving, I'd then stop off for either a pre-made sandwich, crisps, fizzy drink, and cookies, or it would be McDonalds and another latte and a breakfast wrap. I'd rush brunch down, whilst driving, not really tasting anything. That was at least another 1000 calories.

Already I've consumed over half of my daily recommended calories. There was no time to let my food digest. I'm back into the city traffic, I'm speaking on the hands free, and when not on a call my mind is racing thinking about the day ahead. En-route I would hear the ping ping ping ping ping ping from notifications for emails, texts, Whatsapp messages, Facebook messages, and Slack messages. I would answer as many as I could whilst swallowing brunch and lunch down, but there would always be something not answered or dealt with which would nag, nag, nag at me.

I would eventually get to the job, frazzled and bloated. I would rush around dealing with what I had to deal with; in and out of the car, taking calls, dealing with staff, dealing with guests.

Lunchtime would arrive and that would often be a drive thru for my midday fix of comfort food. Another 1000 calories would be consumed. I'm now over my recommended daily calorie allowance, but more importantly, the insulin levels are rising high as are the stress hormones.

The remainder of the day would either ramp up in terms of stress levels caused by any sort of delays, guests turning up early pressuring us for keys, or cleaners deciding that they had to unexpectedly go home early for whatever reason they came up with. My time rushing around would be wholly dependent upon many factors. I was never in charge of that part of my life, but assuming that everything was done and dusted for around 6pm, I'd start my journey home. Usually there would be a call to Amanda who would fill me in on the day's events. That call would last for anything up to an hour as I crawled through rush hour traffic. By now I would be very tired. As I drove home I'd be worrying about the ping ping ping ping from that demanding little computer that I carried around all day. That, along with doing the next day's rosters for the cleaning team would dominate the rest of my evening.

By the time I had reached my home town there was a decision to make. What would be for dinner? Around 7.30pm, with at least an hour's work to do yet, did I really want to cook a meal? Would something to throw in the microwave save time? Or would I phone ahead to our local take out for pizza, or maybe fried chicken, burgers, or kebabs? I can admit now that for that period in my life there would be a mix of meal options, but what always happened was that I would stop off at the supermarket for a bottle of booze. In my mind this was my little treat for all the hard work, and stresses and strains I'd dealt with that day.

So I'd get home, say hi to everyone, pour a large glass of booze which wouldn't touch the sides, and I'd go and start work again. Whatever it was that we ate there would be in excess of 1500 calories consumed. Fast food is fat food. The insulin levels would be high as well due to the amount of added sugar in the processed foods. Then it was time to drop to sleep on the sofa. At least 5000 calories consumed (but not enjoyed) in that one day.

Cortisol - The Stress Hormone

There is another extremely important reason that we must control our stress levels in relation to weight gain and that is cortisol. Cortisol is a steroid hormone which is produce by the adrenals. Cortisol isn't just produced by stress but is also produced by exercise, and by the foods that we eat. Every single cell in our body has a receptor with cortisol in it. This means that if our cortisol levels are too high, or too low, then it affects the cells in every part of our body.

Cortisol can regulate the blood sugar, it can regulate your mood, it can regulate your metabolism, regulate your blood pressure, and it also regulates the water/salt balance in your body. But here is the thing, cortisol in the right amounts can actually trigger and accelerate fat loss. In our bodies is something called hormone sensitive lipase. This is an enzyme that triggers stored fat to release from the tissues of your body and become mobilised in the blood stream. The released fat can then be burned as energy.

This makes sense. When we exercise, the body produces cortisol which calls on fat so that we have energy. This is good, but when cortisol levels are raised for a prolonged period of time then this has the reverse effect on the body. If you have excess cortisol running through your body then you may gain weight, and suffer from mood swings, anxiety, loss of libido, and sleeplessness. I want to share a number of ways in which I believe I have reduced the years of raised cortisol levels which I believe has caused so much of my weight gain:

1. Getting up

Cortisol levels in the blood is naturally higher in the mornings for obvious reasons. We need to get up, prepare for the day ahead, and get moving. We have lots going through our heads about the day ahead, what needs doing, when these things need doing, where we need to be, and when. As the day goes on our cortisol levels tend to reduce. During the evening the cortisol levels are at their lowest as we relax and prepare for bed.

I'm generally an early riser. I set the alarm but rarely need it as I awake around 6am every day. I've noticed a significant difference in my performance and mindset on the days I wake up naturally, as opposed to the rare days when the alarm awakes me. When the alarm wakes me, I turn it off, then drift back to sleep, often waking up later in a panic because I am now late, or now really behind with my schedule. During those days I feel out of sync, I'm a little stressed, I tend to concentrate on negatives, the exercise routine feels arduous, and I usually feel the need to snack with something sweet and comforting.

What I find that really works for me is to get up in good time, potter around, let the cats in, let the dog out, squeeze a lemon for a pint of water, let the birds out and collect the eggs. After checking on my emails and social media, I then get ready to do my morning session whilst listening to an audio book of choice. I come back, feel great, and am ready for the day ahead feeling positive and relaxed.

2. Breakfast

Do I really need breakfast every day? I'll discuss this more in the nutrition section of this book, but as I'm writing about the control of cortisol I think it's worth mentioning. For years I'd get up, put the coffee machine on, have anywhere between 2 - 6 cups by the time I was ready to eat. If I was on the road I'd be consuming large sized, sugared, milky lattes. These would raise my insulin levels through the roof!

Breakfasts at the farm would often consist of bacon, eggs, and buttered toast. Again, this would spike the insulin levels early on in the day which could well send me on an up and down cycle of cravings. What would be far better would be to consume a protein and fat rich breakfast to cut those carbs and feel full for longer, or even better, continue the fast and skip breakfast altogether.

3. Recognise stress

Identifying stressful thinking would also help me keep the cortisol levels down. By recognising stressful thoughts, and then simply writing them down with an action time frame against them, would help. I have learned to brain dump such thoughts at the start of the day. It helps keep the head free to think clearly without undue stress.

Understanding the reasons why stress can cause weight gain explains a lot to me and my relationship with weight and stress over the years. This understanding has definitely focussed my attention to deal with unwanted and often unnecessary stresses.

My Relationship With Food

Another huge and crucial aspect of understanding my relationship with food, is to understand my own psychology. If I could get to the root of why I was overeating then hopefully I could re-align myself. Not just for the weight loss, but my weight management in the future. This would enable me to hopefully succeed with some tough endurance challenge ideas that I had bubbling away in the back of my mind.

For me, food had become a friend, a social pastime, something to alleviate boredom, a comfort in times of negativity, and a treat. For many people, including me, food can become an addiction, or an obsession, and it will obviously determine whether we are healthy or not. Food also dictates the way we think, in far more ways than thinking about what and when to eat.

Eating certain food types changes the chemistry in our brains which in turn can change our behaviour. I was eating a lot of stodgy comfort foods that would initially make me feel better, but the reality was that I actually felt worse afterwards due to lethargy and bloating. This in turn would make me feel short tempered and I would snap at my kids for making a noise and waking me up from my napping on the sofa. Add to that the realisation that what I was eating was very likely going to shorten my life. Not much comfort there.

My lifestyle of rushing around, grabbing fast foods, eating on the move, eating for comfort, eating for treats, eating for convenience by consuming addictive nutrient deficient foods, meant that I kept eating, and eating, and eating. My body was crying out for proper nutrients!

Did you know that an overweight person can be malnourished? Malnourishment has little to do with the quantity of food consumed. A malnourished body can be vitamin and mineral deficient due to poor quality food. The brain increases the appetite hoping to get the much needed vitamins and minerals but is rewarded with a greasy doner kebab or a bowl of ice-cream instead. Can you see the problem here?

Hard Questions and Honest Answers

When I started my fat loss regime I carefully considered the following questions. If you are looking for your own transformation then I would advise you do too.

1. Do I eat when I am bored?
2. Do I comfort eat?
3. Do I love sugary foods?
4. Do I view food as a social occasion?

5. Do I treat myself with food?
6. Do I often fail to plan and prepare my meals?
7. Do I snack in between meals to keep my energy up?
8. Do I often eat late at night?

If the answer to any of these questions is yes then perhaps you need to carefully consider your relationship with food. Think about the types of foods, the quantity of foods, and the timing of the food that you are eating.

Answering these questions with brutal honesty helped me see my own eating habits from a more objective position. Hiding from the truth will serve you with no purpose.

Always Available, Easy To Cook, Processed Food

In my lifetime, and as I write this I have just turned 50, I've witnessed a mammoth increase in availability and promotion of heavily processed fast foods. But at the same time we see little by the way of education on what these foods and drinks actually do to our body, mind, and health.

The supermarkets are crammed with easy to ping foods and there are fast food outlets on almost every street corner. I already knew, as I suggest many other people already know too, that these foods are bad for us. So why do we choose such fattening, processed, nutrient lacking foods? Well, I believe that we learn to eat poor quality food for the following reasons:

1. To save time
2. Early conditioning from TV adverts
3. Easy availability
4. A lack of awareness and education on what effects these foods have on us
5. Addictive additives such as salt and sugar

Bad Eating Habits

Moving to a deeper level, there are other psychological reasons for our bad eating habits. I know that I for one have been very guilty of consuming the wrong foods due to negative emotions such as; annoyance, frustration, boredom, stress, anger, or sadness.

I've illustrated earlier in this chapter how eating would fit around my work and business life. Running my own business which has many moving parts to it with no set hours meant that I had lost any good eating habits learned over the years. This meant that I was disordered in my habits which directly resulted in a detrimental effect on my health and wellbeing. What did that mean for me?

1. Waiting until I was really hungry before having to eat but then eating way too much.
2. Choosing the wrong foods because I was so hungry and needed my 'fix'.
3. Yo-yo dieting every now and again because I disliked how I looked and felt.
4. Starving myself to try and lose weight but having no understanding of how the body works.
5. Getting into the habit of snacking between meals on sweet foods and drinks.
6. Not drinking water. I'd be dehydrated and suffer from regular headaches.

Mindless Eating

Whilst studying the psychology of eating, I learned about a habit that is referred to as 'mindless eating'. This is when we eat whilst doing something else; watching TV, reading, travelling, or chatting. We finish the meal but then realise that we haven't really tasted the food. This is important as it can have a negative impact on your health and weight. I know it did for me.

I would often eat whilst watching the TV every night. Lunch

would either be on the move or whilst working at the computer, or whilst engaging on social media. A common fault of mine was to be concentrating on, or talking about, anything and everything else whilst eating. I'd have little idea if I was full or not, no comprehension if I was overeating or not, and never mind if I was actually chewing the food enough for my poor digestive system.

Eating at set hours is another form of mindless eating. You may sit down to eat at set times such as 7am for breakfast, 1pm for lunch, and 7pm for dinner. It is common for people to sit down at regimented times to eat, even if they are not hungry. It really isn't healthy for your body and for your weight management if you are eating for the sake of it, rather than through real hunger.

Stress and depression, both of which I have suffered with in my weight gain years, is another example of mindless eating. Eating sweet or savoury snacks when I wasn't hungry was typical. This is emotional eating. Food would be fulfilling a purpose other than hunger and providing nourishment.

When I acknowledged what mindless eating was, and that I was a culprit of it, I found the most effective way of dealing with this was to ask myself questions when I thought about starting a meal.

1. Am I really hungry?
2. Have I eaten enough now?
3. Am I eating the rest through greed now?
4. Do I really need that pudding, or do I just want it?

What this discipline does, in time, is to establish mindful eating patterns. The more you think about your food, the more you enjoy it, and the more you will question your food choices as you consciously put it into your mouth.

Cultural Conditioning Around Food

During my studies I learned about the psychology behind how

we learn to deal with food. I found this extremely interesting. To learn the behaviour around food is totally relevant to us a species. In western society we begin our lives drinking only milk whether that is from our mother's breast or from a bottle. Then at around 6 months as we start consuming solid foods, our parents tell us to eat everything up. It is often the case that if we don't want to eat everything up we are scolded and punished. Around this time, we are introduced to sweets, chocolate, fast foods, and processed foods. All these foods are highly rewarding to us. The brain gets a rush from sugar, salt and fat.

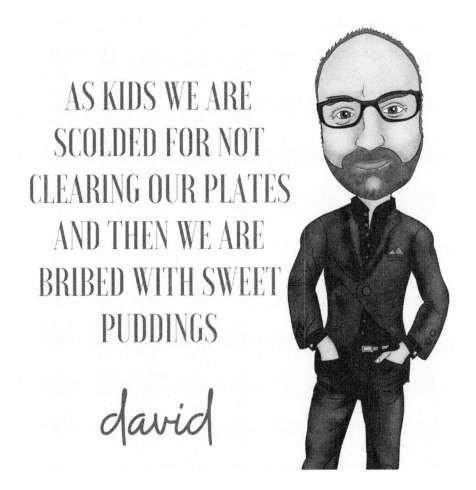

AS KIDS WE ARE SCOLDED FOR NOT CLEARING OUR PLATES AND THEN WE ARE BRIBED WITH SWEET PUDDINGS

david

We are taken out with our parents when they go shopping for groceries. We are promised a chocolate bar (or similar) to sit still, or walk calmly and be good, or we are given a treat whilst being pushed around in the trolley. Chocolate, sweets, crisps, sugary drinks are given to us as a reward for being good. Good children get sweets. Good children get an ice cream. Good children get sugar.

Isn't this a vital area of learning for us? You bet! People often believe that they are addicted to certain foods and those foods often contain lots of sugar. Considering the way in which we are conditioned as youngsters, this could simply be, or at least partly be, emotional addiction. This is called conditioning. As we then get older we begin to find our way in the world and another type of conditioning occurs. This conditioning comes through the effects of society and advertising.

Advertising

We are susceptible to the effects of advertising and so it's very easy to feel not good enough when growing up in those teenage years. We can become very self-conscious, we want to fit in, and we want to be accepted. We see funny, glamorous, attractive and successful people on TV and on social media and we want to be them. But at the same time we are subjected to the power of advertising with the same people tempting us with trendy, sweetened drinks for example. We are psychologically seduced into believing that drinking them will make us happy, fulfilled, cool, socially accepted, and so on. Even healthy! How can over-sweetened energy drinks be healthy?! The advertisers are experts at putting these feelings inside of us. This exposure to psychological manipulation in our pre-teen and teenage years can be extremely damaging. During my studies I came across the following which I want to share.

Ad critic Jean Kilbourne presented to an audience at Harvard T.

H. Chan School of Public Health in March 2015. Kilbourne went on to deconstruct the subconscious messages in food and body image related advertisements and to describe how they create a 'toxic cultural environment' that harms the relationships with what we eat. Kilbourne explained that the average woman encounters 3,000 advertisements every day, and spends a total of two years watching TV commercials in their lifetime. At the centre of many of these ads is an image of an idealised female beauty. Models are slim, light skinned, and can be digitally altered to even more unrealistic body proportions. She went on to say:

> *"Women and girls compare themselves to these images every day. Failure to live up to them is inevitable because they are based on a flawlessness that doesn't exist"*.

This ideal of beauty has become so pervasive that 50% of three to six year old girls worry about their weight.

Advertising creates this disconnect between women, and also men to a lesser extent, and their bodies. It also offers food as a comforter and a proxy for human relationships, Kilbourne went on to explain. She showed images of ads offering chocolate as a substitute for a lover, and cookies presented as a way to get love from your kids. Alongside the chocolate ads were others that shame women for having an appetite for food, Kilbourne gave an example of one that showed a pair of cinnamon buns hanging off a slim model's hips. These images normalise disordered behaviours around food such as bingeing and guilt.

Kilbourne called for a transformation in the way in which we think about food. She said,

> *"The solution to obesity isn't to make girls hate themselves. If we learn to eat healthy, natural, preferably local food with pleasure, and if we exercise with pleasure, our bodies will get to the weight, shape, and size that they were genetically meant to be"*.

There is no doubt in my mind that advertising affects self-esteem and can make children feel unworthy. It is said that three to six year old girls are affected enough by advertising to worry about their own weight. Isn't that absolutely dreadful!?

Emotional Eating

There are so many reasons why we develop a strange relationship with food. Trauma can also cause a lack of appetite which in turn can become anorexia. Poor body image can cause bingeing and vomiting, or taking laxatives. Binge eating and obesity are often related low self-esteem. Food addictions can take over our lives, and our sense.

In my fat gain days I was a culprit of what is called 'emotional eating'. During my studies I learned that the Mayo Clinic describes emotional eating as 'the connection between mood, food, and weight loss'. Emotional eating is consuming food as a way of suppressing, or easing, negative emotions such as stress, anxiety, fear, sadness, loneliness and boredom. For me, issues like divorce, family court, recession, and redundancy, led to negative emotions. These negative emotions led to me to emotional eating and weight gain. Of course some people have the reverse effect and eat less if they are upset in any way, but that wasn't me.

Whatever emotions drive you to overeat, the result is the same. The emotions return and you may feel the additional guilt and end up setting back your weight loss goal. This can lead to a very unhealthy cycle. The emotions trigger overeating, you beat yourself up for ceasing your weight loss program, you feel bad again, so you overeat again.

Dr Jennifer-Kromberg for 'Psychology Today' undertook a deeper study into the reasons people emotionally overeat. She said:

"Most people think emotional eating is due to lack of self-control. However, in my extensive work with eating disorders and disordered eating, I would say that is rarely the case. If emotional eating were a simple issue of discipline, we could easily find this discipline without torturing ourselves over meal plans, paying money for special diets, and constantly obsessing about who is eating what and when, and, of course, no eating disorders".

According to Dr Kromberg, the following five factors contribute to emotional eating:

1. Unawareness - I've been guilty of this. Not being conscious of what or why I'm eating. Therapists call this unconscious eating. This is when you are full up but you still continue to pick at it. I'd do this in the evening whilst eating cheese and crackers.

2. Food as your only pleasure - I'm not sure if this was strictly me as I'd eat and consume alcohol every day too. It seems that people interviewed in relation to this problem would often say that if they didn't binge then they would have nothing to look forward to. Incredibly it is thought that eating sugars and fats release something call opioids in our brains. Opioids are the active ingredients in cocaine, heroin, and other drugs. Considering this, it's hardly a wonder why eating such food as fries and ice cream are so soothing to us.

3. Inability to tolerate difficult feelings - when we are kids we learn to avoid things that don't feel good. We have found that distracting ourselves from difficult feelings are not always in our best interest. Without the ability to tolerate and deal with life's inevitable stresses, we are all very prone to emotional eating.

4. Body hate - this was certainly me for the ten years after I stopped swimming. I hated the way I looked. I couldn't even watch the video recordings of our events. Photographs weren't as bad because as a fat person I learned to position myself in such a way that I didn't look as fat as I actually was. What may sound odd is that hating one's body is a huge factor in emotional eating. Shame, negativity, and hatred rarely inspire people to make long standing positive changes, especially when it comes to our bodies or our sense of self. It has been commonly said that people will stop hating their bodies, but you must stop hating yourself first before you can stop the cycle of emotional eating.

5. Physiology - yet again this was me as I let the stresses and strains of 365 working days a year wear me down. Becoming too hungry or too tired is a great way of putting yourself into a vulnerable state for emotional eating. When the body is tired, it sends strong messages to the brain that you need to eat to provide energy. When we are tired we are less equipped to deal with cravings or urges to eat.

Emotional eating is powerful and is a major reason why I put on so much weight on, as so many people do. To stop the cycle you must commit to reach deep inside yourself to find a place of grit, strength, and determination and then hopefully with understanding what emotional eating is, this problem can be conquered.

Food Addiction

I have rather an addictive personality. When I like something, I really like something. I don't for one minute think I'm in the minority and so thought I should mention it in this book. There is a common ground with all eating disorders. The addictive person moves away from a healthy relationship with food, to an unhealthy relationship with food. The type of disorder, how serious it is, and the combination of habits are entirely per-sonal but the eating disorder itself is defined by a list of action or symptoms for diagnosis. There are lots of reasons why we develop food related behaviours, but the majority of these are psychological.

The single largest problem with food addiction is that it often goes unrecognised. I've always struggled with weight, until recently I never considered food addiction as an issue. I just thought I was a bit greedy.

The two different types of addiction to food are emotional addiction which I have discussed in the previous section of the chapter, and physical addiction which I will expand on now. I have no doubt that I have been addicted to cheese, crackers, crisps (savouries), because for weeks I was craving these evening treats. Cheese contains a protein called casein. When casein is broken down into compounds, these compounds attach to the dopamine receptors in the brain. Now I don't have the cravings. I broke the craving. It can be done.

The other food addiction is chocolate. I don't know if you are like me but sometimes I crave chocolate. As well as sugar and fat, which the brain loves, chocolate contains tryptophan. Tryptophan is an amino acid that is a precursor to serotonin, the happy chemical. Interestingly there are a number of foods, including broccoli, which contain tryptophan so it must be the combination of this with fat and sugar that makes chocolate cravings so common. Again, for the first few weeks of going on this journey I craved the sweet taste of cold chunky chocolate. I'll be honest, now the habit has been broken, I could take it or leave it.

Food addiction is, quite simply, being addicted to junk food in a similar way as drug addicts are addicted to drugs, but obviously less dangerous or life threatening. Food addiction involves the same areas of the brain, the same activated neurotransmitters, and many of the symptoms are identical, just less intense. This is very similar to several other eating disorders, including binge eating, bulimia, compulsive overeating, and having an 'unhealthy' relationship with food. Processed junk foods have a powerful effect on the reward centres of the brain involving brain neurotransmitters like dopamine. This is usually to do with sugar, salt, and fat, all vital to our survival which means our brain is constantly searching for it. Food addiction is not about a lack of willpower, it is caused by the intense dopamine signal 'hijacking' the biochemistry of the brain.

When considering food addiction and whether or not we suffer from food addiction, it is worth noting a number of the most common symptoms. It seems that if you can relate to four or five of these then you likely have a problem with food. If you can relate to six or more (like I was) then you are most likely a food addict.

1. You frequently get cravings for food, even though you might have just finished a meal and you are feeling full.
2. You give in and start eating the food that you have been craving. You then find yourself eating much more than you intended to eat.
3. You have feelings of guilt after eating certain foods that you were craving after.
4. You eat to the point of feeling uncomfortable and bloated after eating food that you craved for.
5. You make up reasons for eating the foods you crave for.
6. You hide the craving foods from other members in the household.
7. In an attempt to stop eating the food you crave for, you attempt to have days off, restrict yourself, and set rules but you always fail.
8. You mask the food cravings from other people.
9. You know that your eating habit is potentially harming you, but you carry on regardless.

It has been found that food addictions are linked with loneliness and the lack of life satisfaction. For me, I wouldn't say for one minute that I have suffered a lack of life satisfaction, but the past decade has had some extremely stressful and testing times which have certainly affected me.

Sugar Addiction

Now is a good time to discuss sugar and how this can very easily cause addiction. For a long time after waking up the first action of the day was to put the coffee machine on. Without any thought at all I would consume up to six coffees. Each coffee would be sugared with two full teaspoons. Later that day I'd consume chocolate, cookies, and cake, all washed down with lashing of sweet tea and fizzy sweet sugary drinks. Early evening I'd crack open the beer, wine, or gin, whiskey, or vodka and drink for the next couple of hours. After dinner there would be often be some form of sweet dessert to top up the day's sugar intake. I was a walking talking snoring sugar filled overweight man. Every day.

1. I'd consume the sugar - I craved it and it made me feel good.
2. My blood sugar levels would spike - dopamine would be released in my brain and mass insulin would be secreted to drop my blood sugar levels.
3. My blood sugar levels would fall rapidly - the now high insulin levels would cause immediate fat storage and my body would now crave the lost 'highs' created by the sugars.
4. I'd then get hungry and want more - the low blood sugar levels would cause increased appetite and further cravings. The cycle is repeated over and over again.

In humans, refined sugar has a drug like effect. It is a very powerful stimulant, and whilst acting as a typical stimulant which gives us highs, it also gives us lows that can cause tiredness, lethargy, and of course more cravings for more sugars. This effect causes mood swings, energy highs and lows, and sugar dependency (hypoglycaemia). In addition to this, fluctuating blood sugar levels can lead to irritability and depression. It can even cause schizophrenic behaviour, menstrual problems, hormonal disturbance, and ulcers. It has even been shown that sugar consumption can affect memory and brain function and that eating too much sugar can give rise to Alzheimer's-like symptoms. It's incredible that we consume so much of this innocent looking white powder.

Of course a very well known risk of high sugar consumption is type 2 diabetes which is usually the result of over eating, under activity and a genetic disposition. Type 2 diabetes is a lifestyle disease which can often be reversed through diet and exercise. Cutting down on sugar stops the insulin spikes, so the pancreas which produces insulin can recover from years of over exertion.

Finally, another effect that this lovely white granulated powder so many of us love spooning into our food and bodies, is that sugar depletes vitamins in the body that we take from quality foods. Sugar not only replaces vitamin rich foods in the diet, it also reduces absorption of crucial vitamins and minerals.

It's pretty terrible when you consider all this, but the great news is that it is possible to break this addictive cycle and I can assure you that I have. No more do I need to be consuming vast amounts of sugar to get me through the day. It is so much better for my body and it feels liberating not to be controlled by this addiction from the moment I wake up, until the moment I go to sleep. So what do we need to consider when breaking this hold sugar has over our mind and body?

The first thing is to have an understanding of what sugar is:

1. Glucose is the actual sugar that we add to tea and coffee and is present in so many refined carbohydrates. The body loves glucose hence why we get the feelings we get when we consume it.
2. Fructose or high fructose corn syrup which is concentrated fruit sugar. Fruit sugar that is in fruit is good because the fibre in the fruit balances out the sugar. How-

ever when fructose is present in a highly refined form,
it overwhelms the body and this may cause problems.

Whilst I am pleased to say that I have broken the sugar cycle,
and now I don't really miss sugar in my food and drinks, I do ac-
knowledge though that this does take some getting used to. Not
spooning heaps of sugar into drinks is one thing, but walking
straight past the refined foods on shop shelves is another. I have
to walk faster! Perhaps always be mindful of the hidden sugar in
refined carbs, ready meals, and junk foods. Leave them there and
save your money. Identify the aisles full of sugar and salt and
avoid them.

I'll tell you how I broke my sugar addiction later on in the book.

Intuitive Eating

A very important aspect change in my lifestyle, and my relationship with food, is what is called intuitive eating. This can
be life changing if done correctly and it takes us right back to
the natural and healthy roots of basic eating habits and wellbeing.

There are only three guidelines to bring intuitive eating into
your own life as I have. These are:

1. Only eat to stop hunger.
2. Stop eating when you are full.
3. No food is bad for you.

Whilst (1) and (2) seem common sense, (3) seems odd considering how we know that refined foods are bad for us. What you
need to remember is that intuitive eating is based on leaving
behind the mental process that has led you to an obsessive or
problem relationship with food in the first place. In order to
achieve this you have to stop labelling foods at all, then stop
treating them like your friend or enemy dependent on the scen-
ario.

The goal of intuitive eating is to only eat when and what your body needs. When you gain this knowledge about yourself then all this will be much easier, and you will naturally and intuitively choose the foods which are high in nutrients.

On the days where I don't fast, I keep my body biologically fed with adequate levels of energy and carbohydrates. If I don't do that then I'm just going to get hungry and start wanting to eat, which will quickly turn into wanting to overeat. If you can learn to honour this first biological signal then you are on your way to re-building trust with yourself and food. I now find myself not wanting the rubbish I used to eat. It's not a conscious thing, I just don't.

What you will also need to do is to call a truce and stop what is known as the 'food fight'. Allow yourself unconditional permission to eat. If you are telling yourself that you shouldn't eat a particular food (but you really want it), then this can lead to intense feelings of deprivation that can lead to intense cravings. These cravings can eventually result in binge eating where you just give in and give up.

When undertaking intuitive eating you should shout NO to any thoughts that may go through your head that say you are being good for eating less calories, or bad because you have had a piece of chocolate cake. I've learned that 'dieting' creates rules that nobody wants to live by. This, in my opinion, is why so many people fail.

Getting to know yourself and accepting your relationship with food is crucial, at least it has been for me. During the initial period of my transformation I kept a journal to help identify what I was doing so naturally. I would ask the following questions:

1. When am I triggered to eat?
2. What am I triggered to eat?

3. Why am I triggered to eat?
4. What am I eating?
5. How do I eat?
6. How does eating make me feel?
7. How do I feel straight after eating?
8. How do I feel 2/3 hours after eating?
9. How do I feel the day after I have eaten?

If you are reading this and you are thinking how tedious, in some respects you are right and I'd agree, but for me this was crucial in understanding my relationship with eating. I didn't do this for long, only a week or so. So it's really not super tedious if you are serious about change.

Journalling Your Food habits

I believe it's worth journalling for a week or so ahead of your transformation. This really helped me understand myself, my reason for eating, and what the foods were doing to my mind and body. It is important to remember that this IS NOT A DIET, this is about self-awareness, so eat what you would normally eat. This is the first stage of the healing process.

Here is a snapshot of one of my journal entries using the same questions above:

1. When am I triggered to eat? *Thursday 10.43am*
2. What am I triggered to eat? *Cheese on toast*
3. Why am I triggered to eat? *Felt starving*
4. What am I eating? *Three slices of brown bread with melted cheddar cheese*
5. How do I eat? *Fast*
6. How does eating make me feel? *Good*
7. How do I feel straight after eating? *As though I want more*
8. How do I feel 2/3 hours after eating? *Hungry again*

9. How do I feel the day after I have eaten? *Sluggish*

That day I hadn't eaten breakfast yet so felt really hungry by 10.30am. I craved something savoury so decided on cheese on toast. I wasn't fasting, and so wasn't in that mindset and routine. I just hadn't planned my eating for the day.

I also learned about 'mental chatter'. Have you ever been assaulted with mental chatter? I mean the endless thoughts that seem to be on a loop that we can't escape from. When we fall into a habit of dysfunctional eating, as I had, the inner voice talks to us about our body shape and how we eat. That voice will constantly attack our self-esteem. It asks us how we dare go out looking like we do. In my case, I got to the stage of not wanting to undress in front of Amanda due to the shame and guilt I felt for looking as I did. The voice also asks why we can't stop eating, why we are such a failure when other people have a control on their health, weight, and fitness, and so it goes on. We need to consider why this inner voice seems so intent on damaging us, as it did in my case.

The negative chatter in my mind was based on conditioning, not facts. What this means is that the negative chatter is based on what is learned from the environment around us, from almost the moment we are born. Everything from critical comments from unthinking parents, to a poor self-image created by the callous system of advertising, has given the inner voice the words it knows will hurt us.

In addition to the repetition, the negative chatter also makes presumptions based on prior learning. An example of this is a negative comment about weight from a thoughtless person and this can have a snowball effect. The inner voice will soon start looking for similar negative evidence to back up this belief. I recall firing a cleaner from our serviced accommodation business. Whilst a Whatsapp message from her calling me a 'fat bastard' was fairly typical of her attitude, it still stuck in my mind.

It wasn't the 'bastard' that stuck in my head, it was the 'fat' that stuck in my head. That example certainly added volume to my inner voice. It didn't even matter that she herself was grossly overweight. She called me 'fat' and I was triggered.

Neuro Linguistic Programming

Finally on getting the head sorted, I have to discuss what I've learned and implemented with Neuro Linguistic Programming (NLP). NLP is a therapy that works towards change for the positive. Whilst NLP is complex, in part it is used to assess and change the memory patterns formed around negative beliefs of the mind. At its core, NLP is a method for replicating excellence, that is excellence in results, excellence in methodology, and excellence in human cognition.

If I was a sports competitor, for example, NLP could be used to model a higher class competitor in the same sport. Modelling what they do, how they do it, and replicate them to improve my results quicker than what it would have taken them to get where they are. That is if I had the time to devote to the sport, if I had total access to watch them perform, if I could interview them, and if they could help me refine my process, then I could conceivably take a lot less time in getting to their levels than it took them. It is possible that I might even become better at teaching the sport than the player I was replicating.

I could potentially then package observations about their skills that they neither could, nor would, have ever concluded on their own. My version of their skills, would arguably have become an NLP based skill. We always teach our mentees to associate with, and get to know and model people who are in a more advanced position than themselves. I knew that if I could, I would need to do the same. Luckily I had a great friend, Pete Rowan, nine years my senior, who was a fitness machine. I could model various aspects of him to help me achieve my goals and challenges.

NLP techniques can be highly effective in the short term. Although that may help the evaluation of the behaviour, learning as much about the therapy would give the best and most effective long lasting results. One of my problems over the fat gain years was giving into my cravings. If you have ever had cravings then I trust that you will agree with me that they can be very strong drive to eat. I know that during the failed 'diets' of the past I'd suffer terribly from cravings and it was those that would ultimately lead me to failure. If I was to lose five stone quickly then I would have to deal with cravings, ideally eliminating them completely.

Food Cravings

Cravings for food are the body signalling that there is a lack of nutrients. For example, chocolate cravings (of which I has previously suffered from more times than I care to remember) may be symptomatic of a magnesium deficiency. Fatty food, carbonated drinks, and alcohol cravings often being a need for extra calcium. Eating a balanced diet of mainly unprocessed foods helped me to alleviate cravings very quickly, so much so that I can't remember the last time I suffered from a craving.

Luckily for me, I learned about the effects of insulin on the body and immediately started intermittent fasting. This meant that I could drop the restrictive dieting that causes cravings. After a week or so the cravings just faded away. If you are reading this and this makes sense to you, I strongly suggest that you consider dropping restrictive dieting, especially if you have some form of compulsive eating. Forbidden food is always so much more desirable. Stop weighing and stop counting. Your body will thank you.

Avoiding sugar-free foods and beverages is very important as they can still trigger cravings for the sugar that they are substituting. This made complete sense to me. During the whole 70lb loss period I haven't had a single 'diet' food or 'diet' drink.

Dealing With Food Cravings

I also learned to ask myself the following questions on the rare occasion that I could feel a craving coming on:

1. Am I really hungry?
2. If the answer to (1) is 'yes' then am I sure that this is hunger and not a craving?
3. Could this feeling be thirst? I would take a drink. This would usually eliminate the feeling.
4. Considering the food I was craving I'd ask myself 'is this what I want'?
5. Considering again and ask myself 'am I really sure this is what I want'?

When asking yourself these questions, it is really important to be honest with yourself. If you over-analyse your answers then you may deny what is really happening within yourself and the whole process may fail.

If my answers to the above questions were no then I would ask myself the following questions:

1. What is it that I really need right now?
2. I'd consider (1) again and answer honestly.
3. What would make me feel better there and then?

By going through the process I would be able to make a considered and educated choice and the craving may have actually gone.

Another way of dealing with a craving is to accept it. Cravings happen, it's usual, it is to be expected and therefore it is important to accept that it is absolutely okay to have them. They're natural. I learned that accepting a craving for what it is, rather than resisting it, lessened the intensity I had suffered from in the past with unsuccessful dieting regimes. I also learned to have internal dialogue to help me deal with unwanted cravings. I would tell myself that it's okay to crave, it's expected, it can be dealt with, it will pass, and I'm in control of this.

In addition to all the above, I learned to focus my attention on how great I felt after overcoming the previously negative feeling of a craving. Cravings don't last and when I'd overcome the craving, and it had well and truly passed, I would feel a sense of achievement. Whereas in the past I would have given in, now I'm stronger, more committed, and ready to get myself fit, lean, and healthy.

Finally, on the topic of this all important diet breaker it was important for me to understand the following. Cravings are probably a signal that the brain has associated eating with pleasure, or with the move away from pain. This means that consuming food and certain drinks becomes a method to modulate feelings and sensations. I didn't want this to happen to me so I learned and practiced. Before I go on it is worth noting that this is powerful and I understood that this should only be used if everything else failed so if used improperly then I may never want to eat the food I was craving for again. I'll explain this step by step process in more detail:

1. What would giving into a craving cost me? I would imagine myself in front of a mirror and think about how I felt seeing myself fat and unhealthy. My internal dialogue would be that of an obese middle aged, unattractive man. I would feel ashamed of the man who was too ashamed to undress in front of his wife.

2. I would choose that image and that would represent what these cravings are costing me.

3. I would then concentrate on sensations, feelings, and further images that these cravings caused in me.

4. I would then concentrate on the foods that I am currently craving. The foods that make me feel bad inside.

5. I would then imagine holding these foods and looking in the mirror with my obese and fast ageing body.

6. I would now welcome the craving for this food and all of the craving sensations that I was feeling.

7. Now I would imagine bringing the food closer to my mouth and feel the consequences of giving in. The fat, obese, unattractive, unfit, version of myself that I was ashamed to show. This image would be made as big as I could in my mind.

8. I would be prepared to repeat this exercise until the craving had passed.

A cautionary note that I had to remember: focus on the craving first, not the food, because the wrong way around could put me off the food forever. That's another eating disorder.

I want to conclude this section of the book by saying that unless the head is in the correct place then a transformation will be really, really tough. The day I locked up our gates for Lockdown, was the day my head locked into doing everything I could to save my health and life. Mindset isn't just important, mindset is crucial.

CHAPTER 4

The Natural Nutrition Network™

T here was no doubt that my dietary choices of the past didn't support my health and wellbeing. Consuming processed foods, fast foods, and refined foods had been directly responsible for my weight problems. I knew that it was crucial to gain a clear understanding on how the body reacts to certain food types.

So What Can I Eat?

Let's face it, this nutrition thing is a maze. We are given so much conflicting advice. How on earth do we know what we should and shouldn't eat?

Don't eat meat.

Do eat meat.

Don't eat too much fish.

Eat plenty of fish.

Don't eat fats.

Do eat fats.

Okay, but which type of fats?

Don't eat carbs.

Restrict your carbs!

Do eat carbs.

Choose your carbs.

Sugar is okay.

Sugar is bad.

Coffee is bad.

Coffee is good!

Which type of coffee is good then?

Tea is good.

Tea is bad.

Restrict tea.

Drink only certain kinds of teas.

Eat lots of fruit.

Don't eat too much fruit.

Drink lots of dairy milk.

Dairy milk is bad for you.

Replace dairy with almond, soya, and nut milk.

But soya is bad for you.

Cheese is good.

Cheese is bad.

Eggs are good.

Eggs are bad.

Restrict your intake of eggs.

Artificially sweetened drinks are good.

Artificially sweetened drinks are bad.

It goes on…

Then you have different diet plans to follow based on excluding foods for ethical as well as health reasons. Are we?

Vegan?

Vegetarian?

Flexitarian?

Ovo-vegetarian?

Lacto-vegetarian?

Lacto-ovo-vegetarian?

Pescatarian?

Ketogenic?

Mediterranean?

Raw food?

South Beach?

Macrobiotic?

Alkaline?

Atkins?

Paleo?

Dukan?

HCG?

Zone?

And then we have the protein battles between meat and plant based diets.

And we hear that the traditional three meals per day plan is the correct way to go!

But then we hear five, six, seven and even eight meals a day are best for weight loss!

But then we hear one meal a day is preferred and intermittent fasting desirable!

But then we hear the experts saying that intermittent fasting isn't good for us!

Then of course we hear don't eat late!
Eat late!

Eat early!

No need to eat early.

Is it any wonder that there is an epidemic of obesity throughout the world with so much conflicting information? When I started out on my mission I decided that I would do my very best to educate myself in regards to nutrition. I needed to design a common sense, sustainable eating routine (I hate the word 'diet') that I could stick to for the long term.

For reference, whilst studying a Diploma in Nutrition, and an Advanced Diploma in Nutrition, the most eye opening book that I read had to be 'The Obesity Code' by Jason Fung MD. This book would completely change my thinking behind the calorie counting theories drummed into me over the past fifty years. To reach my goals, to sustain (and even improve on these goals) I would have to take the most common sense approach for me. I worked on changing my core beliefs around calorie restricted diets, and I would enjoy the process. I knew from old habits that unless the process was enjoyable then I would undoubtedly fail.

Insulin

Before I talk about food I want to touch upon the hormone known as insulin. Insulin has a huge effect on weight gain, on our ability to lose weight, and how it determines whether or not we maintain our weight. That said, I'm not a scientist or a doctor, and so I'm sharing an overview of what I have read and studied, and how I have integrated these learnings into my weight loss regime. The control of insulin levels can be enhanced through nutritional practices as well as intermittent fasting. I'll come back to intermittent fasting later in the book.

When you eat, your insulin levels go up. Insulin is the hormone that tells the body to store fat. When insulin is telling body to store fat it also stops the body from burning fat. This is important to remember, you can't store energy and burn energy at the same time. Any carbohydrates that you consume get converted into glycogen, which are chains of glucose, a type of sugar. Carbohydrates include dairy, fruit, starchy root vegetables, legumes, and sugary processed foods.

When you don't eat your insulin levels fall and your body gets the signal to start drawing on energy reserves. You will pull energy out first from the glycogen (from the carbs) because it is easier than converting the stored fat.

When there is a surplus of energy the energy is stored as fat in the body. The body can draw energy from the fat but it is insulin that allows or restricts that fat energy to be used. What that means is that if you have a lot of insulin then you can't get to the fat to use as energy. Insulin locks away fat. This is why it is extremely important to keep insulin levels down because we need to burn that excess fat away. If our usual subcutaneous fat stores are full, our body starts packing it around our organs in the body cavity. A large waist often indicates large amounts of both types of fat, and insulin resistance.

Insulin sensitivity is the relationship between how much insulin needs to be produced in order to deposit a certain amount of glucose. You are insulin sensitive if a small amount of insulin needs to be secreted to deposit a certain amount of glucose, and insulin resistant if a lot of insulin needs to be secreted to deposit the same amount of glucose. Insulin sensitivity describes how sensitive the body is to the effects of insulin. If you are thought to be insulin sensitive then you will require smaller amounts of insulin to lower the blood glucose levels than someone who has low sensitivity. Having a good sensitivity to insulin is a sign of good health.

Enhancing Insulin Sensitivity and Resistance With Food

There are three main types of insulin sensitivity. These are peripheral insulin sensitivity, hepatic insulin sensitivity, and pancreatic insulin sensitivity.

Insulin sensitivity is seen as good whereas insulin resistance is a major risk for the development of type 2 diabetes.

You can enhance your insulin sensitivity through exercise. It is known that the enhanced insulin sensitivity after exercise is associated with adaptations in skeletal muscles such as increased expression of key proteins such as GLUT4, hexokinasa II, and GD, involved in insulin stimulated glucose metabolism. I know that this is now sounding like a biology lesson, but I believe that it is important to understand the basics on how insulin works.

A person can also enhance their insulin sensitivity through carbohydrate consumption. Insulin sensitivity is at its highest first thing in the morning and also after an exercise session. This is when your body has its lowest muscle and liver glycogen. Therefore the body will be more receptive to absorb the carbohydrates taken on, rather than secreting large amounts of insulin in order to store excess glucose as lipid for another time. As such, when preparing a meal plan with the intention of improving insulin sensitivity, it is important to try and put the bulk of the daily carbohydrates into the first meal of the day, or after exercise.

Consuming the correct foods is the easiest and most effective way of enhancing insulin resistance. Fibrous foods are ideal. It is fibre that slows down the digestion of carbohydrates which means the body gets a steady feed of glucose to use, rather than a large influx of sugar which makes insulin levels peak. Fibre rich foods also tend to have a lower Glycemic Index (GI). This means that these foods cause a slower release of glucose into the bloodstream. This in turns results in lower amounts of insulin to be secreted and the blood sugar in the body remains steady and without significant fluctuations. Trans fats and refined sugar should be completely avoided. Food containing trans fats (biscuits, pastries, ice cream, bread, and cakes) impairs insulin sensitivity.

Enhancing Insulin Resistance with Supplements

Supplements may also be taken to enhance insulin sensitivity such as Green Tea Extract, Chromium and Polyphenols from Cinnamon, N-3 Essential Fatty Acids, White Bean Extract, DHEA, Vitamin D, magnesium. Let's look at how a selection of these effect insulin.

1. **Chromium and Polyphenols from Cinnamon** - scientific studies have suggested the naturally occurring compounds found in chromium polyphenols which are found in cinnamon can increase insulin sensitivity.

2. **Green Tea Extract (GTE)** - GTE can help with insulin sensitivity. Firstly it helps control the inflammatory process that are (partially) responsible for the development of insulin resistance and secondly helps cut down on carbohydrates by block-

ing their digestion and assimilation.

3. **Yacon (Smallanthus sonchifolius)** - this an Andean tuberous root and contains fructoseligosaccharides, insulin, and phenolic compounds. This has a low calorific value and doesn't increase the levels of blood sugar in the body. Studies have shown that Yacon syrup has beneficial effects on obesity and insulin resistance in humans. Long term consumption is believed to have improvements on insulin sensitivity.

4. **Green Coffee Extract** - Green coffee beans are rich in Chlorogenic Aside (CGA) which is a substance with strong antioxidant and anti-inflammatory activity. When roasted the CGA is reduced, along with its properties, and for that reason green coffee is thought to be more beneficial than the normal coffee associated with roasting. The intake of green coffee can prevent weight gain and support weight loss when used with a healthy diet low in fat and refined sugar.

5. **Raspberry Ketones** - Raspberries are a superfood due to their ketones, phytochemical that form the primary aroma compound of red raspberries. In is believed that raspberry ketones affect the production of certain hormones that speed up the body's fat-burning process.

Measuring Insulin Sensitivity

Insulin sensitivity is measured through a method of measuring the skin fold at the shoulder blade. This will give an indication as the whether you are insulin sensitive or insulin resistant. The lower the reading means the more insulin sensitive a person will be, and the better their handling of carbohydrates. If the reading of body fat is below 10 then a person will be classed as insulin tolerant (insulin sensitive). If the reading is higher than 10 then that person is classed as insulin resistant. Back fat is bad.

It is worth repeating, insulin resistance v insulin sensitivity -

insulin resistance and insulin sensitivity are two sides of the same coin. If you have insulin resistance then you have low insulin sensitivity. Conversely, if you are sensitive to insulin then you have low insulin resistance. Whilst insulin resistance is harmful to your heath, as prior noted, insulin sensitivity is beneficial to health. Insulin resistance occurs when the cells stop responding to the insulin hormone. This causes higher insulin and blood sugar levels. This has the potential to cause type 2 diabetes.

The main causes of insulin resistance may be overeating and an increased body fat. Other factors that may cause insulin resistance include a high sugar consumption, inflammation, inactivity and genetics.

It is because of my new appreciation of insulin that I decided to concentrate on following a lifestyle that would control my insulin levels, rather than counting calories. We are told that weight loss is as simple as counting calories, restricting calories, and burning off more calories than we take in. Calories in versus calories out. I have dieted in the past by following the calorie in calorie out theory. Calorie counting is misery. One calorie doesn't have the same nutritional value as another calorie.

Having an understanding of how crucial insulin was to fat storage I next wanted to understand more about metabolism. I had heard about how metabolism can slow down as a person gets older and how having an faster metabolism can help weight loss. This is what I have learned.

Metabolism

Metabolism is the biochemical process that occurs in a living organism (including us humans) to maintain life. It is these biochemical processes that allow us to grow, reproduce, repair damage, and respond to the environment around us. It is metabolism that is responsible to convert what we consume by way of food and drink into energy. It is during this biochemical process that calories (in food and drink) are combined with oxygen to release the energy our bodies need to function. Even when the body is at rest it needs energy for its functions such as breathing, circulating blood, adjusting hormone levels, growing, and repairing.

The number of calories your body uses to carry out the basic functions is known as the basal metabolic rate (BMR) - this is known simply as your metabolism. There are a number of factors that affect someone's basal metabolic rate. These are:

Body size and composition - people with larger bodies, or who have more muscle, will burn more calories.

A person's sex - men usually have less body fat, but more muscle, than women of the same age and weight. This means that men will burn more calories than women.

A person's age - as you get older the amount of muscle tends to decrease and fat accounts for more of a person's weight. This slows down calorie burning.

Energy is needed for our body's basic functions and this requirement remains reasonably consistent and are not easily changed. A person's basal metabolic rate accounts for between 60 - 75% of the calories they burn every day. Then there is nearly 10% energy expenditure whilst eating and digesting. Other normal activities such as exercise and casual movement accounts for between 15 - 30% of daily energy spent.

In additional to your basal metabolic rate, two other factors determine how many calories are burnt each day:

Food processing (thermogenesis) - this is digesting, absorbing, transporting, and storing the food consumed. This accounts for around 10% of the calories used each day.

Physical activity and exercise - is by far the most variable of the factors that determine how many calories we use each day. Doing resistance exercise helps in increasing muscle mass whilst boosting overall calorie burning. Exercising on a daily basis will mean that I would be maximising my energy burn.

Natural Metabolism Boosters

There is also what are termed natural metabolism boosters, a couple of examples to note are:

Thyroid supporters: Thyroid hormones control the body's metabolism. A dysfunction of the thyroid gland, especially the under-functioning of the gland, can lead to weight gain. Sea plants and seaweed like kelp can help the thyroid gland function normally. The reason is their high content of iodine which is a trace mineral vital for good thyroid function.

Thermogenic phytochemical: Epigallocatechin gallate is a type of phytochemical that is part of the catechises family and is found in green and black teas. In smaller amounts it is also found in java beans, raspberries, and cocoa. These have been associated with weight reduction through thermogenesis and metabolism speed up.

Water

Another hugely important factor in the fat loss attack is the consistent consumption of water. When you are actively working to lose weight, water helps as it acts as a weight-loss aid because it can help you eat less. Drinking water provides hydration without unwanted calories. Simply replacing those fizzy and sweetened drinks that spike insulin with fresh drinking water will have huge effects on your body and health.

Drinking water also helps with any feelings of hunger you might get when cutting out those snacks or when fasting. During my period of fat loss I would consistently consume around 2 - 4 litres of fresh water per day. I must say that replacing the sweet drinks with water took lot of getting used to. However, I believe that this simple and cheap act was a major contributor to my results, and there are also huge health benefits to drinking water on a consistent basis. I'll note just a few because when I reached my goal, I will need to continue these great habits to maintain a good quality healthy lifestyle.

Water serving as a lubricant - water is necessary for digestion. Water in saliva helps when chewing and swallowing. Water also lubricates joints and cartilages allowing them to move with fluidity. When the body is dehydrated water is taken away from the joints which can cause joint, knee, and back pain which in time can lead to injuries and arthritis.

Water regulates the body temperature - the body can control over heating through perspiration from sweat glands in the skin which evaporated and produces a cooling effect.

Water removes harmful toxins from the body - this occurs in many different ways. Water flushes waste and toxins from the body through urination and perspiration. Water also helps with constipation and helps bowel movements, ensuring waste is removed quickly and regular before it becomes poisonous in the body. Waste builds up when dehydration becomes a regular occurrence which in turn can cause headaches, toxicity and illness. Drinking the correct amount of water also lessens the burden on the kidney and liver by flushing out waste products. I suffered for years with regular headaches. Little did I appreciate how little water I was taken onboard.

Water transports valuable nutrients to the body - blood is composed of 92% water which carries nutrients and oxygen throughout the body. The nutrients consumed through the food we consume are broken down in the digestive system where they become water soluble. Water allows the nutrients to pass through capillaries within the intestinal walls to the blood and circulatory system where the nutrients and oxygen is distributed to all the cells and organs.

Water helps with the prevention of diseases - water is extremely important in the prevention of diseases. It is believed that by drinking eight glasses of water per day can decrease the risk of colon cancer by 45%, bladder cancer by 50%, and can potentially reduce the risk of breast cancer. This list is not exhaustive. Why would we not engage in such a simple act of drinking water when there is scientific proof that water helps prevent such life threatening disease?

Water is crucial for transporting blood plasma - the movement of water within the cellular systems transport blood plasma which is made up of 92% water. It is the blood plasma that plays a critical role in buffering the body's pH, circulating antibodies from the immune system, and regulating osmotic balance which helps maintain proper body temperature.

Water helps maintain blood pressure - a lack of water can cause a thickening of the blood which can in turn cause higher blood pressure.

Water helps maximise physical performance - drinking plenty of water during physical activity is absolutely crucial. During exercise you may perspire anywhere between 6 - 10% of your body weight. Clearly this water loss needs to be replaced.

Water may boost metabolism - another extremely important contributor to weight loss and extremely important to start the day by drinking fresh water.

When I get up in the morning the first thing I do is to drink a pint of water. When I'm not fasting I'll squeeze a fresh lemon to make lemon water. If I don't carry out this simple act then wow, do I feel the difference. If I don't consume a consistent amount of water during the day I can feel myself becoming dehydrated.

I can recognise hydration now, something I couldn't do before my health kick. Drinking water has been a friend to me over this period in so many ways.

Superfoods

When starting out on this transformation, I thought it necessary to try and understand superfoods. If I was to maximise the effect of healthy eating then I'd want to be eating the best food I possibly could. So what are superfoods?

Superfoods are defined by the Food and Agricultural Organisation as those foods which are intended to be consumed as part of the normal diet and that contain biologically active components which offer the potential of enhanced health or reduced risk of disease. Superfoods are foods with naturally occurring bioactive substances (e.g. probiotics) and synthesised food ingredients to traditional foods (e.g. probiotics). Superfoods can play a big role in weight reduction as they can encourage alkalinity and also detox our bodies. It made complete sense for me to consider integrating superfoods at every opportunity I could.

I learned that a properly alkalised body has an ideal pH so it functions better and has a faster metabolism. A detoxed body has the ability to easily remove harmful and pathogenic toxins. Some superfood examples include spirulina, chlorella, wheatgrass juice, garlic, beets, celery and cruciferous vegetables such as cauliflower, cabbage, kale and sprouts.

Since March I always have plenty of the following superfoods in our kitchen:

Proteins:

Salmon (wild)
Lean red grass-fed meat
Omega 3-rich eggs

Greek yoghurt
Whey protein supplements
Tuna (line caught)

Vegetables and Fruit:

Spinach
Asparagus
Cruciferous vegetables (cauliflower, cabbage, broccoli)
Mixed berries (raspberries, cherries, blueberries)
Apples

Carbohydrates (other carbs):

Brown rice
Sweet potato
Whole nuts (gluten free)

Good fats:

Mixed nuts
Nut butters (almond and cashew)
Extra virgin olive oil
Fish oil
Flax seed

Drinks:

Green tea
Nutrient rich smoothies using the ingredients listed above.

Herbs and Spices

Nature assists us to achieve permanent and efficient weight loss by providing us with a variety of natural ingredients such as herbs, spices, minerals, and vitamins. These compounds can reduce the need for restrictive diets and harmful weight loss drugs.

One of the most important natural products are herbs. A herb is defined as any plant with leaves, seeds, or flowers used for flavouring foods, medicine, or perfume. Herbal remedies have been used for treatment of human aliments for thousands of years. They possess a long history with the first known book about herbal healing dating back to 2700 BC in China. Herbs, fresh or dry, in foods or teas can significantly assist with weight loss. Again, it seems bonkers not to add herbs into your daily meal plan at every opportunity. Why on earth would we not?

Another really important group when considering health and weight loss is spice. Spices are natural food additives that have been used as flavouring, seasoning, and colouring agents. Spices have also been used as preservatives throughout the world for thousands of years. Spices have been widely used for weight loss purposes due to their anti-adipogenic and thermogenic actions. I'll explain this:

Anti-adipogenic spices contain phytochemical (phenolic acids) which have anti-adipogenic effects in the body. A great example is curcumin which is found in turmeric. As one of the main functions of adipocytes is the lipid storage, an anti-adipogenic phytochemical like curcumin helps reduce body fat mass and body weight by preventing fat storage.

Thermogenic spices, capsaicin and capsiate, active components in red and chilli peppers are known for boosting metabolism and for their ability to enhance fat oxidation. Fat oxidation is the breakdown of fatty acids. I'll say again, why not integrate these spices into our daily food intake?

Vitamins

Before starting off on this journey I had read somewhere that vitamins can help you lose weight. Wanting to take every advantage I could I looked further into this and I found that the answer was YES, they can!

Being overweight and obese has been linked with a deficiency of some types of vitamins. If we increase their consumption, and reverse that deficiency we can speed up the fat burning process and reduce weight from our bodies.

Vitamin A

Retinal, or Vitamin A, plays an important role in regulating body weight, Body Mass Index (BMI) and waist and hip circumference. The richest plant sources of vitamin A are paprika, cayenne, chilli peppers, carrots, and sweet potatoes.

Vitamin C

Ascorbic acid, or vitamin C, is inversely related to body mass. People with enough vitamin levels burn 30% more fat during a moderate exercise compared to people who have low levels of vitamin C, thus, a vitamin C deficiency may mean resistance to body fat loss.

Studies show that whilst the majority of people think that they consume enough amounts of vitamin C, in America the majority of adults are estimated to be deficient. The reason for this is because vitamin C is easily destroyed during the cooking process.

If you smoke then absorption of vitamin C is hindered which leads to inadequate levels in the body.

The highest source of vitamin C is chilli peppers. One green chilli pepper can provide 182% of your recommended daily intake of vitamin C. Other rich sources include bell peppers, fresh herbs like thyme and parsley, kiwi fruit, broccoli, and guavas.

I squeeze fresh lemon juice in my water on a daily basis which not only livens up the water, and makes it taste refreshing, but is a great way of keeping my vitamin levels up.

Vitamin D

Vitamin D is really important for weight loss. There are studies that strongly associate low vitamin D with abdominal fat. Vitamin D causes fat cells to become more metabolically active which helps the body burn more fat.

Mushrooms are the best vegetarian source of vitamin D and the top animal source is from fish, such as cod liver oil and oily fish such as salmon, mackerel, sardines, and tuna.

We now consume mushrooms every day and salmon and tuna account for three meals per week. Garlic mushrooms is a favourite as the dish takes in umpteen superfoods which are rich in nutrients. I've added some recipes later on in my book.

Minerals

As well as vitamins, I have also studied minerals. I never really knew what minerals were but it turns out that they can make some really positive differences. It doesn't matter how small a difference a mineral can make, what is important is the overall effect of all these small changes in the food that we eat.

Chromium

This mineral reduces body fat and decreases appetite. Chromium can also support normal cholesterol and triglyceride levels, can help to maintain normal blood sugar and insulin levels, and contribute to better overall health.

Sources of chromium include liver, fish, milk, and whole grains. Chromium-rich herbs include catnip, horsetail, and nettle. See, your stoned cat isn't so daft.

Calcium

Calcium is of course commonly known for healthy bones and teeth. However, a range of studies suggest that calcium may also lead to a lower prevalence of being overweight, obese, and insulin resistant. Calcium influences energy balance and regulates fat metabolism in the adipocytes (fat cells). It is therefore important to consume the correct amounts of calcium rich foods to help us lose fat faster.

Examples of high calcium food sources include dark leafy vegetables such as spinach, okra, broccoli, watercress, as well as almonds, fish and dairy products.

Amino Acids

Also known as the building block of protein, amino acids can significantly aid both weight and fat loss. The most important weight loss amino acids are considered to be:

Lysine which is an amino acid that plays an important role in the production of carnitine. This is a chemical compound responsible for the conversion of fat cells into energy and helping lower body fat and cholesterol. The best food sources of lysine are red meat, fish, poultry eggs, parmesan cheese, nuts, and legumes.

Tyrosine has the ability to improve mood swings. Improving mental health can contribute to higher levels of motivation and happiness, something that can help in the treatment of obesity. High tyrosine foods include pork, fish, beef, chicken, tofu, beans, cheese, milk, nuts, seeds, and whole grains.

Phenylethylamine also has the ability to treat mood problems and depression. A naturally occurring chemical found in the body, it can also be taken orally to improve athletic performance as well as attention. It's probably no surprise that this amino acid can be found in chocolate, cheese, sherry, and wine. Mmmmm, phenylethylamine.

Now Put All That Into A Meal Planner!

We've discussed the confusion of conflicting studies and reports and the contradictory advice from the experts. We've looked at why calorie based diets are misleading. We've discovered that restrictive diets are difficult to follow and and doomed to medium term failure. I may have told you that I don't like the most healthy food at all, vegetables! I had to put it all together into something easy to follow, and still be healthy at the same time.

The following weekly schedule isn't a set in stone schedule. It is a typical week that changed slightly in terms of timings and meals choice depending on what I was doing and what the family fancied that day.

It is worth noting that this was the schedule when I was fasting every other day for between 22-24 hours.

	BREAKFAST	LUNCH	DINNER	SIDE DISH	DESSERT
MON	Granola, banana, lemon water, smoothie	Cheese, mushroom, spinach omelette	Sirloin steak, poached eggs with mushrooms, spinach, and cashew nuts in mustard	Boiled baby potatoes	FAST Water and green tea
TUE	FAST Water and black coffee	FAST Water and black coffee	Thai chicken red curry.	Brown basmati rice, boiled	Strawberries and raspberries in cream
WED	Granola, banana, lemon water, smoothie	Garlic mushrooms on sour bread toast	Lemon and black pepper king prawns	Brown basmati rice, boiled	FAST Water and green tea
THU	FAST Water and black coffee	FAST Water and black coffee	Pan seared tuna, mushrooms, spinach, two poached eggs	Boiled baby potatoes	Fresh fruit selection
FRI	Eggs Benedict and sour bread toast, lemon water, smoothie	Cheese, mushroom, spinach omelette	Mediterranean Chicken with Roasted Vegetables	Boiled baby potatoes	FAST Water and green tea
SAT	FAST Water and black coffee	FAST Water and black coffee	Baked salmon, mushrooms, green beans	Boiled baby potatoes	Water melon
SUN	Granola, banana, smoothie, lemon water	3 poached eggs on sour bread toast	Lamb Nihari	Brown basmati rice, boiled	FAST Water and green tea

MEAL IDEAS

I thought that it would be good to include a few recipes of my favourite dishes in this book which I have loved to eat, have supported my mission, and are packed with nutrients.

MEAL 1

Garlic mushrooms on sourdough bread

Preparation and cooking time - less than 10 minutes.

Amanda and I love garlic mushrooms so let me share how I cook them. This is really easy.

Ingredients

Chestnut mushrooms
Fresh garlic
Olive oil
Fresh parsley
Fresh sage
Salt and pepper
Sourdough bread.

So how do we cook?

1. Take the fresh garlic and chop into really small pieces.

2. Next I chop the parsley and sage up.

3. Take the mushrooms and chop these into quarters.

4. Generously pour virgin olive oil into a pan and apply the heat.

5. When the oil is hot, throw the garlic in and stir for a

couple of minutes.

6. Throw the parsley and sage in and stir.

7. Now throw the mushrooms in and stir until cooked. Depending upon the heat and the size of your mushrooms cooking times will be around 4-5 minutes.

8. Take the sourdough bread, either toast on a skillet type pan or simply toast.

9. When the mushrooms are cooked, and the bread is lightly brown, tip your garlic mushrooms onto the toasted bread and let the oil soak in.

10. Enjoy.

This meal is packed with superfoods - mushrooms, virgin olive oil, sage, parsley, and garlic. We often eat this meal as a small lunch but I will often increase the portion size to serve for dinner. It's a great meal if you are wanting to cut down on meat consumption.

MEAL 2

Veggie omelette

Preparation and cooking time - less than 10 minutes.

Guys, please, please, please, if you are going to buy eggs, please buy free range and not eggs from the hell hole battery farms, also known as caged birds. Amanda and I have rescued many a hen from these disgusting hell holes and these poor birds are walking (if they can walk) skeletons. It's horrific and I beg you not to support this industry.

Okay, so let's get cooking. I use either hen, duck, or goose egg for my omelettes and to be honest there isn't a great deal of difference when put into an omelette, apart from goose eggs are huge!

Ingredients

3x duck eggs (or 2x chicken eggs, or 1x goose egg)
Cheddar cheese or vegan cheese
Mushrooms
Spinach
Parsley
Fresh garlic
Salt and pepper
Olive oil

So how do we cook?

1. Grab your eggs, crack them, and pour into a cup.

2. Add a pinch of salt and a pinch of pepper.

3. Mix really well.

4. Slice a couple of medium sized mushrooms up.

5. Grab a handful of organic baby spinach.

6. Cut off half a handful of parsley off the parsley plant.

7. Chop up three cloves of garlic.

8. Grate the cheese. Grate as much as you want.

9. Grab a flat bottom pan and add some olive oil.

10. Turn the heat on until hot, but not spitting hot.

11. Throw the chopped up garlic into the pan and stir.

12. Throw the mushrooms, parsley, and spinach in the pan and stir until cooking. Depending on size of the mushrooms, and heat, around 4 minutes.

13. In a separate pan drizzle some olive oil into a pan and heat on a low temperature.

14. Pour the mixed eggs into the pan and add the grated cheese.

15. Make sure the eggs don't stick to the bottom of the pan.

16. Add the cooked vegetables then when consistency allows flip one half of the omelette over the other.

17. Cook until the eggs are cooked but don't overcook.

18. Serve

We love omelette for a protein rich, super food crammed, veggie dish. Of course if you want to add meat to this then great, we tend not to as we use this meal as an enjoyable way of cutting down on the meat consumption. The great thing about omelette is that you can pretty much add what you want for variation.

MEAL 3

*Steak, eggs, with mushrooms
and spinach in mustard*

Preparation and cooking time - less than 30 minutes.

One of my treat meals and a great protein based meal after a good exercise session. I usually go for sirloin, then either fillet or rib eye. Cooking steaks vary depending on personal preference. For me, I prefer a medium to rare steak as I love the taste and texture.

Ingredients

Steak
2x eggs
Brown basmati rice
Mushrooms
Fresh spinach
Olive oil
Cashew nuts

So how do we cook?

1. Pour around one cup of brown basmati rice per person into pan. Rinse the rice then add water. There should be around 10mm of clear water above the level of the rice. Add a little salt and a touch of olive oil to the water.

2. Apply full heat to the pan and boil for around 5 minutes.

3. Cover the pan with a lid and apply a low heat for around 10 minutes.

4. After 10 minutes turn the heat off and allow the rice to sit for around 15 minutes.

5. Remove the steak from any packaging and allow it to sit at room temperate for at least five minutes.

6. Apply olive oil to both sides of the steak and then season to your taste.

7. Apply heat to a pan or griddle. The pan should be very hot. Don't apply oil to the pan, you have applied it to the raw steak.

8. When the pan is hot put your steak in. Assuming that the steak is around an inch thick, leave the steak cooking on one side for around a minute. After one minute turn the steak and allow the other side to cook. This will seal the steak.

9. Depending upon how long you like your steak will depend on how long you cook it. A minute each side is perfect for me.

10. When you are happy take your steak out and cover it with a foil for around five minutes. This will allow your steak to settle. Remember that the steak will still continue to cook as there is still heat in it.

11. Whilst you are cooking your steak prepare your mushrooms, spinach and cashew nuts in mustard.

12. Put the mushrooms into a pan of butter and English mustard and cook for around 3 minutes. Then apply the spinach and cashews nuts. Stir thoroughly and cook for around a further two to three minutes.

13. As you are cooking your mushrooms boil a small pan of water for your poached eggs.

14. When the pan is boiling add your eggs and leave for around 3 minutes. If you prefer them harder then leave for a little longer.

15. Your rice, vegetables, eggs, and steak should now be perfectly cooked. Put them on a plate and enjoy a protein rich, super food rich dish to help those recovering muscles maximise growth.

This is a really simple dish to prepare and cook. I would usually cook this after a heavier exercise session to get as much protein into the body as I possibly can.

MEAL 4

*Lemon, black pepper, and garlic
king prawns*

Preparation and cooking time - less than 15 minutes

We love this seafood dish which is a great source of nutrients. Really easy to cook and super quick.

Ingredients

King prawns, virgin olive oil, salt, course ground pepper, fresh garlic, vegetable stock, butter, parsley fresh lemon, pak choi, noodles.

So how do we cook?

1. Put virgin olive oil in a flat bottom pan and apply heat (medium heat).

2. Chop the fresh garlic and throw it into the hot pan.

3. Stir and make sure the garlic doesn't brown.

4. Throw your king prawns into the pan and cook. Don't overcook. When the prawns turn pink take them out and place on a side dish.

5. In the same pan put some fresh garlic and parsley and fry.

6. Stir and before the garlic goes brown add the vegetable

stock. Add pepper and salt and stir.

7. Add four teaspoons of butter. Add one at a time.

8. In an additional pan add olive oil, garlic, black pepper, and stir.

9. In the additional pan add the pak choi and toss for around 3 - 4 minutes.

10. In the original pan add the king prawns for 1 minute and stir.

11. Add grated lemon zest and freshly squeezed lemon juice to the pan.

12. Add the noodles in with the pak choi and stir until cooked.

13. Take your plate, add the noodles and pak choi.

14. Add the king prawns and the sauce. Then enjoy.

A really tasty and healthy dish and an alternative from meat.

MEAL 5

*Fresh tuna, baby new potatoes
and vegetables*

Preparation and cooking time - less than 40 minutes.

We love this dish and personally the pan seared method of cooking the tuna steaks is my absolute favourite. I love tuna with boiled baby potatoes and at least two vegetables. Of course the choice of vegetables can vary but my personal favourites are mushrooms, and fresh asparagus.

Ingredients - fresh tuna steak, virgin olive oil, baby potatoes, mushrooms, fresh asparagus, salt, pepper, coriander seeds, lemon, and fennel seeds.

So how do we cook?

1. Cut the tuna steak into steaks around 20mm deep.

2. Crush and mix the salt, pepper, coriander and fennel seeds.

3. Add the seasoning to both sides of the tuna steak.

4. Apply olive oil to both sides of the tuna steak.

5. Bring a pan of water to the boil and add the potatoes. Add a little salt for taste.

6. Prepare the mushrooms, add butter, English mustard,

and pepper.

7. When the vegetables are five minutes away from ready heat the pan to receive the tuna steak.

8. Bring the heat to medium hot and put the tuna in.

9. Let the tuna cook for around 90 seconds to 120 seconds to make sure the steak is seared.

10. Add a little olive oil and turn the steak.

11. Cook for 90 seconds to 120 seconds and bring out. The tuna shouldn't be over cooked.

12. Squeeze the lemon onto the tuna steak and serve.

A great protein rich, nutrient dense, dish that can be served in many different ways. I'm not a lover of salad but tuna goes great with various types of salad.

MEAL 6

Scrambled Eggs With Salmon

Preparation and cooking time - less than 10 minutes.

A super protein rich, tasty, easy, quick meal. A great choice for breakfast or lunch.

Ingredients - 3 eggs, 1 tsp olive oil, 100grams cooked salmon, cut into thin slices, parsley leaves (to garnish), 2 tsp fresh lemon juice, salt and pepper.

So how do we cook?

1. Crack your eggs and mix in a cup.

2. Add the seasoning.

3. Dress the salmon slices with lemon juice.

4. Warm the olive oil in a large saucepan on a medium heat then add the mixed eggs.

5. Stir the eggs to break up the texture of the cooking eggs. When cooked serve on the plate.

6. Add the salmon, parsley, and serve.

MEAL 7

Mini breakfast pizzas

Preparation and cooking time - less than 20 minutes.

A really fun and super nutrient rich breakfast treat. I cook this meal when I have some time I the mornings, usually at weekends.

Ingredients

3x eggs
2x Portobello mushrooms
3x cherry tomatoes
30 grams low fat shredded cheese
1/2 tsp dried oregano
1 tbsp olive oil
Ground black pepper and salt.

So how do we cook?

1. Heat the oven to 350F (177C)

2. Remove the stem and scrape out the gills of the mushrooms.

3. Crack an egg on the top.

4. Drizzle the olive oil, add a little pepper (to suit taste), salt and oregano and cook for around 15 minutes.

MEAL 8

Spicy Beef Salad

Preparation and cooking time - less than 10 minutes.

A really tasty, fast, nutrient rich meal perfect for lunch. Easy to make and take if you are out and about for the day.

<u>Ingredients</u>

1x lettuce leaf
Lean beef cut into strips
1x large shredded carrot
2 tsp fresh lime juice
1 tsp chilli flakes
1 tsp chilli sauce
1 tbsp olive oil
1/2 tsp garlic powder
1 tbsp fresh chopped basil
Salt and pepper to taste.

1. Warm the olive oil over a medium heat.

2. Add the garlic, chilli flakes, chilli sauce, and beef.

3. Sauté the beef for only 2 to 3 minutes then leave to cool.

4. Add all the ingredients (except the lettuce) into a bowl.

5. On the serving plate add the lettuce and fill it with the salad.

6. Drizzle with lime juice, sprinkle with some salt and pepper then serve.

MEAL 9

Greek Style Chicken Salad

Preparation and cooking time - less than 15 minutes.

A super nutrient packed lunch which is super-fast, tasty, and can be prepared and taken on the move.

<u>Ingredients</u>

1x roast chicken breast
1/4 cup of goat cheese
1/2 chopped onion
1/2 red pepper cut into strips
5-6 black olives
1 medium sized chopped tomato
Rocket leaves
2 tsp olive oil
1 tsp balsamic vinegar
Salt and pepper.

So how do we cook?

1. Add the ingredients into a large salad bowl.

2. Combine with chicken strips.

3. Add olive oil and balsamic, season with salt and pepper. Serve.

MEAL 10

Chicken and Feta Cheese Burgers

Preparation and cooking time - less than 30 minutes.

A fun, super tasty, nutrient packed meal that is perfect for lunch or dinner. Really easy too.

<u>Ingredients</u>

500grams lean minced chicken (or turkey)
1/2tsp of your favourite mustard
1tsp vinegar,
2 tsp tofu crumbs
1/3 cup tomato sauce
1/2 tsp garlic powder
1/2 tsp mint
1/2 tsp oregano
1x egg
60 grams low-fat goat cheese
1 tsp olive oil
1/2 cup fat-free chicken or vegetable broth
1 cup lettuce.

So how do we cook?

1. Mix the ingredients in a bowl (except the feta cheese).

2. Refrigerate the mixture for 20 minutes. Then remove and form the burgers. Open a hole with your finger in

each burger and then add some feta cheese.

3. Add the burgers in a grill pan together with 1 tsp of olive oil and cook each side for two minutes.

4. Add the broth to the pan and allow the burgers to be cooked thoroughly.

5. Serve with salad.

MEAL 11

*Mediterranean Chicken with
Roasted Vegetables*

Preparation and cooking time - less than 90 minutes.

A really easy, tasty, and super healthy dinner.

<u>Ingredients</u>

1 free range chicken
Juice from 1 lemon
1 tsp oregano
1 tsp thyme
2 tsp olive oil
1 crushed garlic clove
1 medium carrot
1 yellow pepper
1 medium eggplant
Salt and pepper to taste
Water

So how do we cook?

1. Preheat the oven to 390F (200C)

2. Wash and cut the vegetables. Drizzle with 1 tbsp of olive oil and put them into the centre of a roasting tray with garlic.

3. Place the chicken on top of the vegetables, drizzle with lemon juice and the remainder of the oil, then season with salt, pepper, and oregano.

4. Add 1/2 cup of water to the roasting tray and place into the preheated oven.

5. Cook for around 80 minutes then serve.

SMOOTHIES

The Fernley Tropical

Ingredients (made for two)

210g banana
210g pineapple
210g mango
100g vanilla whey powder
600ml coconut milk.
Ice

The Fernley Red

Ingredients (made for two)

130g strawberries
130g blackberries
130g raspberries
100g strawberry whey powder
600ml coconut milk
Ice

Fernley Cocco

Ingredients

Milk
Peanut butter

Chocolate whey powder
Dark cocoa powder,
Frozen banana
Ice

Avocado Smoothie

Ingredients

1/4 avocado
1 scoop vanilla whey protein
1/2 cup raw spinach
1 cup coconut water

Super Green Smoothie

Ingredients

1/3 apple
1 scoop vanilla whey powder
1/4 cup celery slices
1/4 cup cucumber slices
1 cup coconut water

CHAPTER 5

The Free Fasting Formula™

T his is a game changer and if you are considering a transformation of your own, then intermittent fasting is well worth learning about. I didn't start fasting when I set off on my transformation, I only started a few weeks in. Until that point I had seen reasonable weight loss but nothing compared with what was to come.

This is a very short chapter, but it is probably the most important one.

Fasting Isn't A Fad

Intermittent fasting is the controlled, voluntary abstinence from the consumption of foods for a given period. It is as simple as that, and we aren't starving, we are fasting. There seems to be a misconception that intermittent fasting is a new concept but it's not. Hippocrates, the father of Western medicine, believed fasting enabled the body to heal itself. He said that our food should be our medicine and our medicine should be our food. He went on to say that to eat when we are sick, is to feed our sickness.

Benjamin Franklin, one of the greatest minds in history said that the best of all medicines was resting and fasting. Mahatma Gandhi said fasting cleanses the mind, body, and soul. Jesus Christ said Satan and his plagues may be cast out only by fasting and prayer.

Buddhist monks fast every day. The Muslim faith believes in fasting. People all over the world fast on a regular basis and have done so for thousands of years. Muslims from all around the world will fast from sun up to sun down for an entire month for Ramadan.

Our bodies are designed to fast. When we are sick we often don't want to eat. This comes naturally to us. Animals are exactly the same. This is a very natural process. For centuries people have fasted to cleanse the body and cleanse the soul.

Fasting For Health

I have learned that in addition to the incredible fat loss results intermittent fasting would deliver for me, there were also huge additional health benefits. Medical experts and scientists have documented that intermittent fasting is deeply beneficial for heart disease, type 2 diabetes, cancer, and liver disease. For these reasons alone, I have made the decision that fasting will be a part of my life long after the weight loss goals have been achieved. Other incredible benefits of fasting include, autophagy, a rise in ketones, a rise in stem cells, and hormone optimisation. Fasting also resets microbiome, and DNA.

When I first considered fasting I really had to think about whether or not I could do this. I really dislike the feeling of hunger. Feelings of hunger took me back to the failed 'diets' of the past, so I spoke to friends who were fasting to ask how they managed it. They all said that they really believed that they couldn't practice fasting too, but they did, and here is the thing, as I mention above, millions of people fast every day and have for thousands of years. If they can do it then why couldn't I do it too?

Now of course there are people, companies, and organisations who don't want you to fast. Who are these? The manufacturers, producers, fast food chains, and all of their connected commercial businesses don't want you to fast because there is no money in it for them. This is a really important point. Fasting. Doesn't. Cost. Anything. It's free! No shakes, no powders, no pills, no supplements of any sort to pay for.

Incredibly, since Amanda and I have been fasting, and coupled with more conscious eating, our monthly household shopping bills (which would include the booze) have gone from around £900 per month for the four of us (and animals) to between £450 - £550 per month. This simple change in lifestyle has saved us around £5400 per year. It's incredible!

Fasting To Save Time

We haven't just saved money from our grocery bills, we have also saved a huge amount of time. Time that I can spend on my business, my family, and myself. Fasting means shopping for less food, so quicker trips to the supermarket. It means not having to break off from working, or keeping fit, to start preparing and cooking a meal. Fasting reduces the time needed to clean up and put away in the kitchen.

I have seen a huge time saving in my life as the shopper and cook in my family. I want to take a moment to break this down. If you fast every other day like I do then you will miss breakfast and lunch 3.5 days per week. This means that I don't have to shop, prepare, cook, and clean up after up to seven meals per week. I'd take a guess that I spend around an hour of my life delivering, consuming, and clearing up after each meal. That adds up to a total of 365 hours won back over the period of a year. That is a lot of time to spend with my family, dedicate to my business, keep fit, play sport, or just relax.

Fasting To Lose Fat

So how does intermittent fasting help you lose fat? Considering that I am not a scientist, or a doctor, I'm only going to touch on this in this book. This is a huge subject and there are far more expert people than me to explain this if you want to research further.

Intermittent fasting works to keep the insulin levels in the body low which means that when your body is using energy, the suppression of insulin allows the body to draw on the fat stores in the body. We really should have at least a very basic understanding of how insulin works and that includes understanding what insulin resistance is (it's bad). I've already discussed insulin earlier in this book, but I'm not going to apologise for talking about it again because insulin is the key to weight loss and weight gain so it's well worth repeating.

You have to control the levels of insulin. Insulin is the hormonal mediator which dictates where energy is stored. If insulin is high then the insulin is going to direct all that energy towards your fat stores. So for example, you cut the fat off your meat to reduce the calorific value of your meal, but this has no effect on the level of insulin. This means that the energy from the food you are consuming will be directed to your fat stores by the higher insulin levels in the body.

A common belief, and one that I certainly shared, was that switching sugary drinks for low calorie sweetened drinks would stop or slow weight gain. Again, whilst it may be true that there will be a lesser amount of calories consumed by choosing 'diet' type drinks in place of sugary drinks, studies show that there is absolutely no benefit in fat loss because both types of drink spike the insulin levels. When these insulin levels are spiked, the energy is directed to the fat stores by the insulin. Diet drinks don't help diets. Diet drinks will sabotage your diets.

I would urge you to research further the effects of insulin on the body. You will understand how counting the calories will not provide you with a sustained healthy weight loss programme for the medium and long term. Calorie counting only works in the short term, and that is until your body readjusts your metabolism and learns to use less calories. That means that as you cut your calorie consumption, your daily expenditure of energy will also go down.

NO FAD DIETS
NO COUNTING CALORIES
NO SUPPLEMENTS
NO GYM
NO SURGERY
NO TRAINER

david

If you cut your calories by around 25% then your basal metabolism will go down by around 25%. In other words, if you simply take in less, your body will respond by burning less (your metabolism). What will then happen is that as you start to consume more calories, or you aren't exercising as much and thus burning as much energy, then you will start to regain the weight because your metabolism has dropped and you will put on more weight.

So this is the fallacy with calories in and calories out. The key isn't about how much energy you put into your body, it is about where that energy is directed to when it comes in. However with fasting we see that whilst the weight comes down, the basal metabolic rate is maintained. In fact it is likely to be increased from where you started. This is because as the hormone insulin goes down, there are other hormones that go up and that is how the basal metabolic rate is maintained. Hormones not calories.

Don't forget that your body automatically stores excess energy as fat reserves. These reserves are used for energy for if and when you haven't any energy coming in. But artificially increased insulin will block the body's access to those fat stores. If the brain wants more energy it will tell you that you are hungry or thirsty. Just remember that your brain doesn't know the difference between sugar and sweetener and often your thirst is actually a need for sugar. By controlling your insulin levels you are allowing those fat stores to be used as they were intended. You know those diets that suggest you should eat 5, 6, 7 or even 8 times a day? Hello insulin spikes!

Ghrelin

It is also very important that we understand hunger and how we deal with it. Ghrelin is known as the growth hormone and we should have at least a very basic understand on how ghrelin works. Ghrelin is based in the stomach, and it increases hunger.

When we don't eat, ghrelin spikes around breakfast, lunch and dinner. That means at those traditional meal times we get the feelings of hunger, but what happens if we don't eat at those meal times? Ghrelin doesn't keep going up. It actually comes back down meaning that we lose those temporary feelings of hunger. At lunch time, the hunger hormone rises typically around 1pm but then by around 4pm it will have come back down to similar levels as it would have been if we had eaten something. The same happens in the evening. Ghrelin goes up around 6pm but then two or three hours later it goes back to around the levels it would have been if we would have eaten dinner. So hunger doesn't grow and grow and grow. It comes in expected waves and if you can ride out those waves then fasting is very manageable. Another interesting fact is that ghrelin is higher during calorie restricted diets, compared to alternate day intermittent fasting. It is hardly any wonder why those calorie restricted diets fail so consistently.

Managing hunger waves

So I'd like to share how I have managed my hunger levels. It's really simple. By expecting the predicted waves I know that they will come and I know that they will pass. This means that when the hunger waves start I will drink black coffee and/or water in the mornings and green tea and/or water in the afternoons. Both green tea and coffee (not decaffeinated) can help suppress ghrelin. Whilst I haven't been a lover of black coffee or green tea in the past, when I am fasting both are very welcome. Both help with the hunger waves until the ghrelin subsides back to normal.

In addition to managing the hunger waves, by fasting every other day the mind knows that the end of the fast is never too far away. It's not like starving. It's temporary. That understanding has been a huge mindset plus factor for me. The time really does pass quickly and you soon get very used to it.

As already discussed, calorie restricted diets tend to increase our hunger and decrease our metabolism. This means that your weight loss either plateaus or you give up, and put the same weight back on. Through fasting, and drinking water, green tea, and black coffee our hunger is managed and our metabolism stays the same. We're eating less, but we are allowing our fat stores to be used as energy, so we lose weight. Ghrelin is a hormone we want to suppress but leptin is a hormone we want to wake up.

Leptin

Leptin lives in fat cells. It monitors how big the cells are and it tells our brain, the hypothalamus to be precise, that the fat cells are big enough now thank you very much so please stop asking for more fat.

It sounds as though leptin could be a very good friend to us. But unfortunately, due to our overeating, the brain stops listening to leptin and we become leptin resistant. Leptin works in a very similar way to insulin and they work together. The easiest way to reset our leptin hormone and become sensitive to it, is to reduce the fat. The best way to reduce the fat is to burn it. The best way to burn it is to stop blocking the fat burning process with insulin. Cut the sugar. Cut the sugary drinks, cut the sugary food, and remember to cut the artificial sweeteners too.

You can't reduce your fat cells by eating less fat. You need healthy fats, otherwise known as natural fats to function, but you ought to avoid the processed trans fats. Full fat foods will sate your hunger quicker and make you feel full for longer, so some of these are good in a healthy diet. Enjoy tasty butter and bin the fake butter and be guilt free. Low fat foods usually have less taste, so to combat this the food manufacturers add sugar. Low fat = high sugar. But it's not real sugar, its usually fake sugar to make you feel better and it tastes the same anyway. But we now know that sugar and fake sugar increase insulin and insulin stops fat stores from being used as energy. The leptin in the fat cells are crying "No more fat!" but your brain is not listening anymore. Help leptin out, and increase your leptin sensitivity, by reducing the insulin. Your waist line will thank you.

But the loose skin!

One of the biggest fears about losing a lot of weight quickly is the possibility of loose baggy skin that has to be surgically removed. All that hard work to lose weight but you have to tuck your belly away into your waistband and hide it all with a loose top. It's so sad. You can get weight loss surgery on the NHS if you qualify, but so many people have to either live with the folds of saggy skin or they have to raise their own funds to do the additional surgery. Is there anything we can do to prevent, or reduce, the risk of baggy saggy stretched skin?

Did you know that you are only around 7-10 years old? Your cells have a lifespan. Your cells are dying every day, but the good news is that your body is replacing the dead cells with new cells. Phew, but it begs the question 'So, where do the old dead cells go?'

Good question. The answer is autophagy (*awe-toff-a-gee*). Autophagy means self eating, auto means self and phagy means eating. What on earth does *that* mean? It means that the body will use the dead cells as energy and recycle them into producing new cells. Various parts of your body, usually the most important parts are recycled fairly quickly. Your liver can repair itself in 30 days. Other parts up to 7-10 years. Your skin, like any other part of your body, is just a collection of cells. Your excess skin is an unwanted cell bank ready to be recycled and reused to repair or replace other cells in your body. So why do people with extreme weight loss have all this excess skin? Quite simply, their body has never been in a state of autophagy.

Autophagy doesn't happen all of the time. Autophagy only works when the body is in a fasted state and only after 18-20 hours. So in theory you can turn autophagy on, to help reuse your old skin cells and prevent saggy skin. The good news is that autophagy can also break down and reuse all sorts of unwanted cells including ageing cells and malignant cells. Fasting has been shown to reduce the size of known tumours. Isn't this amazing?

Fasting for at least 18-20 hours isn't easy, but it gets easier and now that I understood ghrelin and knew that the fast had an end time I found it easier to go through with it. I decided to fast for 22 hours every other day so that my weekly food intake wasn't dramatically reduced, but I got the benefits of autophagy. I'm very pleased to say that I don't have any baggy skin anywhere after losing 5 stone in just 4 months. It could be good genes and super stretchy skin but it could have been the intermittent fasting.

I'll end this section by going back to my opening statement. I noted that the results I had been seeing prior to practicing fasting were nothing like what was to come. What do I mean? Until I practised fasting I had been losing between 2-3lbs each week. That was fine, it was heading in the right direction. But when I started intermittent fasting that weight loss dramatically increased to between 6-7lbs per week for a period of 3 to 4 weeks. It was crazy. I couldn't believe the scales each week. The results were dramatic, and I wasn't hungry, or fed up.

Too much weight loss, too fast, is not good for you, they say. Don't lose more than 2lb a week because any more than that is not sustainable, they say. If you are calorie counting then yes, I would agree, but, if you are still eating well, and your metabolism is happy and not worried, then why can't very overweight people lose more?

It has to be said that fasting is not an excuse to keep eating sweets, chocolate, cake and pastries. When you fast and get used to that feeling that can only be described as 'clean', you don't want those foods. What do I mean by clean? Well, you stop feeling bloated. You stop feeling sluggish. You feel a mental clarity as well as a lack of indigestion. Your meals naturally get smaller. You want to eat fresh whole foods. I even started eating vegetables.

You will find that the volume of food diminishes but the quality of your food improves. Instead of stodge, you start to eat foods filled with vitamins and minerals and your body will thank you. Because you are eating less, you can spend a bit more on quality food. Treat yourself to the best steak. Try that weird named fish. Sample something you have never tried before.

I've lost 5 stone in just 4 months and I can say that I feel absolutely fine. In fact I feel better than fine, I feel tremendous. I have not felt any negative issues whatsoever in losing that quantity of fat so quickly.

Intermittent fasting will be a part of my lifestyle moving forward. I feel the difference this brings to my health and well-being and I encourage you to consider whether this is right for you.

CHAPTER 6

The Easy Exercise Explainer™

Ten years of progressive weight gain. Ten years in a sedentary lifestyle. 2.3 litres of gin every week. Sugar by the bucket full. Over eating on junk food, with a high heart rate, high blood pressure, and weak muscles, meant starting out on a fitness campaign had to be considered very carefully.

I probably should have consulted with my doctor but this was Lockdown, and doctors' waiting rooms are a good place to catch all sorts of nasties at the best of times. I took my chances.

My renewed love for getting fit and active, and having great fun at the same time, has opened up a world which I never thought I would revisit. A new world that involves running 10km each week, training for marathons, climbing mountains, and training for a triathlon that has been voted one of the toughest in the world. But when I started my fat loss campaign none of that was in my mind. I could barely walk up an incline without bending over, and puffing and panting. My fitness campaign had to start very slowly, with some thought and planning.

For a moment I considered hiring a fitness coach. There is no doubt that there are guys who know their way round a gymnasium blindfolded. They look fantastic, and they know all the theory inside out, but I wondered how many understand the mindset of a middle aged person. Most of them have never been middle-aged and only a few of them may have been overweight at some point. How could they understand me? A person who carries years of stress, both life and business, years of alcohol abuse, obese, and has developed eating disorders?

I don't know, maybe they do, but in my humble opinion there is a difference between having experienced the foregoing personally and really helping someone make the life changes that they need to. I decided that I wouldn't be paying someone who hadn't been in similar shoes to mine. I had enough experience, having been extremely fit in early life, and I had Pete in my corner who had a lifetime of fitness experience behind him and was there as a pal supporting and offering guidance.

Just Start Moving

Health clubs and gyms were shutting due to Lockdown so they weren't an option. At over 19 stone, with stiff joints, running wasn't an option. Swimming pools were shut so swimming wasn't an option. My resting heart rate was between 85-90 bpm so high intensity interval training wasn't an option. All I had at my disposal was a 10kg kettlebell, a dust covered rowing machine, and a pair of Crocs. I soon replaced the Crocs with walking boots. Surely the common sense approach was to just start moving. Moving slowly but moving consistently.

I knew that to improve and then maintain my fitness, any exercise regime would need to be enjoyable. If I started a daily routine with a feeling of dread then it wouldn't last. It would fail within a matter of weeks, more likely it would fail in just a few days.

On the 25 March 2020, when the decision was made to sort myself out, I decided that the very best exercise that I could possible start doing was walking. I'm lucky, I live in a gorgeous place up in the South Pennine moorland. It made total sense to put my Crocs on, pick a route, and move. I grabbed my son Jack and told him to be up bright and early because tomorrow he was going to be my training buddy. He was as thrilled as any other 18 year old lad who loves his bed and computer would be. We would walk to the bottom of our fields, down the dirt path, into the valley, up the other side, and back down the road to the farm in a circular route. This wasn't exciting, it wasn't ground breaking, but it was a start. It would be the start of a routine. It would be a bench mark to push forward on. It would get my heart pumping, my blood circulating, my lungs breathing in super fresh air, exercise my legs and core muscles, and make me feel generally better about myself.

As we were now entering Lockdown and time was available to us, I considered whether I could actually build two sessions into my day? One session in the morning, and one session in the afternoon/evening? Yes, I decided to brush off the rowing machine and the session would be a very modest 15 minute session. Just to start moving again.

Day 1

The first day of my campaign arrived and so did exercise session one. Jack and I set off and walked for 33 minutes. Part way, whilst climbing an incline, I found myself bent over puffing and panting for breath. Whilst shocked at how unfit I was, this wasn't actually a bad thing. I was really exercising my body. I could feel my lungs, my heart, and my muscles working. I had made the start. I eventually arrived back home and I felt great. It was scary really how unfit I had become, but at the same time I was relieved that I knew I could tackle this poor health before the body had failed in some way with something chronic. The afternoon session was extremely modest on the rowing machine, but again, I was moving. I had started, I felt positive, and tomorrow I would add a little more. Just a little but there would be progress.

Making Progress

Over the next few days I kept moving and every day I increased the walking and the rowing. Not a lot, just enough to say I had achieved more than yesterday. I focused my mind on this positive daily progress. In the meantime I dusted off the kettlebell, watched a few YouTube videos on how to use them and then alternated some resistance work in with the cardio from the rowing machine.

The exercise progressed to an hour long walk in the morning and then over 30 minutes rowing in the afternoon with some kettlebell exercises thrown in. I was starting to feel some level of fitness returning and perhaps just as important, probably more important, I was loving this. My mind was focused, and whilst the world was going mad with coronavirus I was in charge of this element of my life.

My weight was coming off but I was still heavy. I could now handle the hour's walk in the morning but I was itching to move faster. I started to mix some jogging in with the walking but I was struggling, I just wasn't quite ready yet. I was quickly putting myself into an anaerobic state which was stressing my body and I was starting to not look forward to going out in the morning. Running at this time was not right for me yet, but what else could I do?

A long time ago I had a weight lifting machine that I had never used. Not wanting to throw it away, I still had the loose 5kg weights in our utility room. Why not grab one of the kids' old rucksacks, throw two weights in, and carry that? This extra 10kg would help with increased energy burn, increased leg and core workout, and importantly continue to push regular progression. Walking was increasing my metabolism and I was losing weight. Surely this added weight would accelerate the losses I was already enjoying by burning more energy? It made enough logical sense to me.

Seeing A Difference In My Body

The next few weeks would be spent hiking around on the hills with weights in the morning for anything between 60 - 90 minutes. In the evening I extended both the time spent rowing and the simple resistance training, and I was enjoying it.

I was loving the progress. I was loving feeling how the body was getting back to a level of fitness. I was loving the fat loss, and I was loving seeing my body gradually changing shape, as my jeans became looser and looser. I was also really enjoying the opportunity of some 'me time' whilst I was exercising, by listening to audio books which would educate and inspire me. I was improving my health as well as improving my knowledge and mindset in one go. I really loved this.

As the fat dropped off and my strength and stamina increased, I weirdly found myself wanting to push myself harder. This push would of course be a daily push through the exercise sessions, but also I'd set myself challenges. Physically gruelling challenges which would really test me.

Challenges like The National Three Peaks 24 hour Challenge which in March 2020 would be a ridiculous proposition because I was so unfit and heavy. Training for that which would include Scafell Pike (the highest mountain in England), Snowdon (the highest mountain in Wales), and the famous Helvellyn (the third highest mountain in England) which is a real test of endurance and nerve.

I also decided to tackle the Yorkshire Three Peaks Challenge which is a non-stop push over 24.5 miles with a combined elevation of 5200ft. The three peaks in Yorkshire aren't the highest but unlike the National, there is no opportunity for rest and a nap between climbs. I'll tell you more about these challenges in the journal section of this book.

Seeing A Difference In My Mindset

As my fitness returned, I was also starting to see huge changes in my mindset and outlook. I was able to relax, and I started to feel younger. It's difficult to put into words but I felt vibrant. I was experiencing more energy and more pride in my appearance. It was with this mindset, and loving the sense of pride these achievements gave me, that I decided to sign up for the Manchester Marathon.

Why not? The Manchester Marathon had been postponed from April 2020 to October 2020 due to Covid so why not take the opportunity to tackle a marathon in six months time? I knew that this challenge would only serve to help me push harder and with more motivation to take my health, fitness, and wellbeing way beyond the initial goal of the 5 stone weight loss. Sadly the Manchester Marathon was postponed again but my new Facebook friend, David, who is part of our Facebook group (Fit For Business) suggested that I might want to have a go at the 'Hell of a Hill Marathon' in November.

So, again, why not! I registered and started training. It was with this new mindset, and a nagging itch to push the body and mind as far as I can, that I also registered for the Brutal Triathlon in Snowdonia in September 2021. A swim in the cold water of Llyn Padarn, then cycling around the mountains of Snowdonia, and then a run up and down Mount Snowdon. I must need my head testing!

When I thought about the fitness side of this transformation I knew that if I was to carry out a daily exercise with no real interest, goal, ambition, or excitement attached to it then I stood a chance of failure. I remembered my swimming days and the drive and determination that got me up at 5am nearly every day to be in the pool even on wet and cold winter mornings. That determination was driven by my desire to be as good as I could be at swimming. I needed some form of competition to keep that commitment going for the many years I swam. If I just turned up to the weights room and cardio machine every day I really don't think that it would have lasted as long as I did. I would have got bored. Competing against someone, even if they don't know about it, gave me an edge and a purpose.

Several years on and I felt the same about competition and having goals and ambitions. My friend Pete, nine years my senior, could leave me standing when climbing a mountain. He has fitness built into him after decades of endurance and strength training. I wholly respected that, but I didn't want to lag behind a moment more than I had to. Neither did I just want to walk/hike/run around the area where I lived. I wanted to take on challenges that tested me and interested me. This would encourage me to go out at 6am even when it was raining, to do an hour on the rowing machine when I really didn't fancy it, and to handle the stresses of day to day business life which can so easily throw you off track. I wanted to get back into some form of sport and I wanted some form of competition. As the next few weeks went by, my focus would move from just weight loss towards pushing myself to new challenges that the old, fat, overweight me could only dream about.

4 Months And 5 Stone Later

Four months later I am now five stone lighter. I am fitter, slimmer, and my clothes are hanging off me. After years of buying the last of the XXXL clothes on the rail I can now choose what I like from the M section. I love M. Rather than having to go to Next, just because they have shirts in my size, I can now browse TKMaxx and find some designer bargains that I love and make me feel great. Shopping for clothes is now a pleasure rather than a bucket full of cold embarrassment and shame.

I now want to see what an ex-fat middle aged bloke can do in the rest of a one year window. Where will this fitness journey take me? I intend to write a second book which will focus on part two of my transformation. That book will concentrate more heavily on the mindset and the more advanced fitness. This section of this book is about the simple steps that I took to drop the weight and get myself back into a good level of fitness.

I was talking to a friend of mine a few weeks ago who had recently suffered a heart attack. He had clearly taken this huge shock very seriously and so had started to try and get fit. We talked about what I did to get my fitness back but his feeling was that walking wasn't enough. I totally understood what he was saying but when I explained exactly how walking was working for me, that it was just the beginning of the progression, he saw it's validity. He had felt that walking was a cop out. He thought that the only way to get fit was to run, and he was worried because he knew he wasn't up to it, and didn't want to over-exert himself into another heart attack. After our talk he realised that walking was just the start and the rest would come in time as his fitness levels and enjoyment increased.

You see, getting fit again isn't about going mad in the gym and then walking around like the Tin Man for a week. It's not about stressing the body out so much that you hike up those stress hormones levels which don't help at all with fat loss. It isn't about stressing yourself out that much that you dread the next session and then find excuses to avoid the exercise. It isn't about doing the things you don't enjoy. It isn't about being bored to death. Neither is it doing pointless exercises that will not show any benefit.

To clarify that last point: I see videos from fitness experts talking about how to turn belly fat into muscle by doing crunches and other repetitive core exercises. How utterly ridiculous! What is the point of struggling by doing crushes, leg ups, planks, or whatever other super-duper core exercises for the muscle to be hidden by a layer of fat? Also don't the experts who talk of 'no pain, no gain' understand anything about cortisol and its effects on the body's ability to burn fat? Why do we see muscle bound experts telling us to carry out exercise that nobody except trained gymnasts can do? It's mad! It's mad because it sets us up for failure time after time, and it's not fair.

We are all different. We are at different ages, we have different health challenges, we have different goals, and we have different lifestyles. I would strongly recommend getting checked out by a qualified health care professional before setting out on your fitness journey. When you start exercising take some time to consider what you can do, what you enjoy, how much time you have, and what you want to achieve. Choose your advice and guidance very carefully and if possible connect with someone who has ideally been through the same challenges you face rather than someone who is far removed from where you are and has perhaps has only ever lived in a gym. This is your health. Choose your support very carefully.

Timing of exercise sessions was also incredibly important during this period. Firstly, I knew that I felt at my best and most motivated in the mornings. I have always been an early riser so getting up, checking my emails and social media, then getting ready and going out suited me. I could be out and back in before the day really got started. Exercising first thing was also great timing because I would probably be around 12 hours into a fast, and my ghrelin would be demanding breakfast.

Exercising whilst in a fasted state helps accelerate the burn of stubborn fat. The growth hormones peak due to the fasted state, which helps accelerate muscle growth. Exercising in the late afternoon at around 21 hours into a fast would produced even more accelerated results. Exercising in the morning would also help to kick start the metabolism early for the day. I wanted the body to be burning as much energy as reasonably possible throughout the course of each and every day. So if you are designing your transformation please consider what are the best times for you to maximise effect, maintain enjoyment, and avoid as much disruption as possible to your normal day. We are all guilty of saying that we are too busy to exercise and keep fit. Really? In a period of 24 hours I find it really difficult to believe now that someone can't find an hour, even 45 minutes, to dedicate to their greatest asset.

> There is a saying - *If you don't make time for your wellness, you will be forced to make time for your illness* - I'll add to that - *choose wisely, and choose timely.*

And finally, I believe that it is important to note that when losing weight, the split between nutrition and exercise doesn't offer a 50/50 result. Clearly I cannot measure this exactly but I'd suggest from my experience over the past few months that the result is weighted around 70/30 in favour of nutrition. What this means is that whilst exercise is of course very important, it is the concentration on nutrition that must take preference. There is absolutely no point in my mind of eating poorly, drinking too much, and then flogging yourself on a running machine.

NO AMOUNT OF TRAINING WOULD COMPENSATE FOR A BAD DIET AND ALCOHOL

david

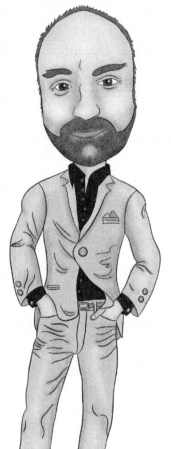

Simply put, **you will never out train a bad diet**. Get the nutrition right, set yourself a realistic and sustainable (and enjoyable!) fitness programme, enjoy the process and keep going.

The next chapter is my journal. After a few days I felt that I needed to journal my exercise, my diet and my mindset. It was there to help me see how far I had come and I think it may help you too. If you are considering starting an exercise and nutrition regime I encourage you to start journalling for the same reasons.

CHAPTER 7

The Journal

26 March 2020

Day one. So decision made and today was the first day of action. I got up early, around 6am, and put the coffee machine on. I love coffee and although the plan is to drop the milk and the sugar, and moderate the amount of coffee I consume, that isn't my focus today. The plan was to get out this morning and start walking. The plan for this afternoon was to get onto the rowing machine and see how long I could last.

I have learned that consuming water is important for the fat loss and also my general health. I drank a pint of water before the coffee to hydrate my body after the night's sleep. I've not done this for years. I've been a coffee-holic and of course coffee dehydrates you. Dehydration on top of dehydration!

The walk today was great but it highlighted just how dreadfully unfit I have become. Jack and I walked a circuit which took us out of the farm and down the adjacent pathway, down into the valley at the bottom of our fields, across the river, up the steep embankment and then back home. I timed the walk at 33 minutes which was okay, it was a start. I was totally knackered trying to drag myself up the valley side. Jack was up at the top, no problems at all, whilst I was bent over, half way up, panting for breath and with my heart pounding out of my chest.

The afternoon session on the rowing machine lasted a short 17 minutes which felt a lot longer. I was puffing and panting, my heart was racing, my back was aching, but at least I have started. 17 minutes is 17 minutes longer than yesterday and tomorrow I'll try to push to 18 minutes. My goal is to be at least pushing to 30 minutes within the next couple of weeks. If I could do that, and also extend the morning outdoor sessions, then I will be getting a decent level of exercise.

In my earlier years my daily exercise would rarely exceed an hour. An hour a day had put me in great shape so if I could get myself to at least an hour a day as soon as possible then I would be on my way.

The first steps to an improved nutrition regime also started today.

- I drank around 6 pints of our spring water throughout the day.

- I had fruit and granola for breakfast

- Lunch was a cheese, mushroom and spinach omelette.

- For dinner I swapped meat for fish and had a wonderful fresh piece of tuna steak cooked in virgin olive oil. To accompany the tuna I boiled baby potatoes, and a mix of sautéed mushrooms and spinach in English mustard.

I'm feeling terrific tonight. I've made decision, I have my goal, and I've started. The alarm is set for 6.30am tomorrow morning and the plan is to extend the morning walk/hike to around 45 minutes. I want to get to that minimum one hour per day as quickly as possible.

27 March 2020

I'm buzzing tonight as I write this. This morning Jack and I pushed on and walked across the moors for a full hour. We started off on the circuit from yesterday but then pressed on that bit further. Getting back home I really felt as though I had made a huge step forward in my determination to do this.

This afternoon's rowing session also went to plan. I pushed for that extra 60 seconds on the machine, and whilst that may not seem like a lot, it was a push further than yesterday which is always positive. A bonus which I hadn't planned for was to locate and dust off my 10kg kettle bell and do two sets of curls. This is weird. My arm muscles aren't used to this and I really struggled. I'm going to start introducing some resistance training in and around the rowing machine sessions.

With regards to the kettle bell resistance work, I have to be mindful that until I start seeing some major fat loss then any muscle that I build will be covered in fat. What that means is that I know, no matter how many weights I lift, until the fat is lost I won't see the benefit. If I don't see the benefit then I am liable to get disheartened. So the kettlebell exercises are just to get used to lifting the weight, and not to start seeing muscle anytime soon.

A good, positive day again with the nutrition improvements.

No snacking between meals. No snacking after dinner. Lots of fresh water, and a huge reduction on the coffee intake. Where I would normally have around six cups of white sugary coffee, I have halved that.

- I had fruit and granola for breakfast.

- Lunch was a cheese, mushroom and spinach omelette.

- Dinner was king prawn in oyster sauce with mushrooms and cashew nuts.

Again, I am making a few changes whilst still enjoying one of my most favourite meals. I've swapped white basmati rice for brown basmati rice. I've eliminated the rubbish carbohydrates, and I've swapped meat for seafood.

Again, I'm feeling great as I write this journal entry. I've pushed into day 2, I've stuck to the plan, and even increased my daily goal. The mindset is absolutely in the right place.

30 March 2020

Today was a really great push forward. I've started mixing the morning hike with a jog (on the flat and downhill) and I've increased my hike to a steeper climb. As we are in Lockdown I've set up a circuit around the farm and into the valley at the bottom of the fields. Each circuit takes around 20 minutes and it's quite steep. This is a real test of the legs going uphill, and downhill for that matter. As much as this is a great session, I cannot complete one circuit without stopping at least twice. The great thing is that I have a tough routine (for me at this time) and I have lots to work on.

The nutrition regime over the past few days has been great. I have no desire to snack in between meals and the head is completely in the right place. We are increasing our fish intake to three nights per week and have reduced bacon and sausages.

Nutrition today was water intake as soon as I got up. Water throughout the day.

- Granola and banana for breakfast.

- Poached eggs with cheese on toast for lunch.

- Salmon, baby potatoes, mushrooms, spinach (in English mustard) and two poached eggs for dinner.

Today's exercise was the new circuits in the morning. A lesser time than the gentler walk I started, but much harder. In the afternoon I did the rowing machine session and am delighted to say that I managed to push this to 20 minutes. There was a midway stop for a breather, but then I carried on to complete the 20 minutes. This is way ahead of where I expected to be. Happy!

6 April 2020

Over the past few days I've seen a very slight, but consistent improvement in my ability to get around the morning circuit. The hills are still killing me, but I'm not stopping as much as I did. I'm really pleased with the progress.

I'm also pleased to note that I'm maintaining my new no snacking rule. This really isn't bothering me whatsoever, not as much as I thought it would. I really think that drinking pints of water throughout the day is eliminating this previous desire to keep eating.

The nutritional intake has also continued to be healthy. I haven't consumed any refined carbohydrates at all, and I'm delighted to say that haven't missed them.

Nutrition today was:

- Granola and banana for breakfast.
- Poached duck eggs on sour bread toast for lunch.
- Seasoned chicken, brown rice, mushrooms, baby sweet-corn for dinner.
- I've consumed around 7 pints of water during the day.

Exercise was 3 circuits around the fields this morning followed by 25 minutes on the rowing machine. I'm now pushing towards the 30 minute target goal.

10 April 2020

It was Friday weigh day today. I'm delighted to note that I've lost 3lb from last week's weigh day. I'm happy with that. At the moment, my concentration has just been to integrate some very simple steps into my lifestyle, that being consistent exercise, cutting snacks, avoiding processed foods, and eating more whole foods.

Since the last journal entry I'm delighted to report that there has been no slipping on snacks or consuming the usual junk foods. I've exercised every day and eaten only whole foods and drank lots of water. I'm really enjoying my meals and so I have absolutely no feelings of being on 'diet'. I'm not restricting anything. No weighing food. No counting calories. I'm just making better choices.

Nutrition today was:

- Granola and blueberries for breakfast.

- Chicken and feta cheese burgers for lunch.

- I made a chicken tikka curry with brown rice and cashew nuts for dinner.

Again, I have loved everything I have eaten today and have no 'diet' calorie restriction, deprived feelings whatsoever.

Exercise was the 3 circuits this morning. I'm maintaining the same distance at the moment. I'm still finding the hike tough going and so my focus is on consistency rather than pushing too hard too soon. This afternoon, I did some resistance training using my 10kg kettlebell.

17 April 2020

I haven't journaled for a week because the routine has been very much the same. I am thrilled to note that I haven't deviated from any of the new lifestyle choices that I put into place.

The exercise is going well as I've been able to push that bit harder on each session. I'm still doing the same 3 circuits but I've added some slow running onto the end. I'm absolutely shattered when I've completed the sessions but getting into the shower feels wonderful. I'm then set up for the day ahead knowing that I have achieved something meaningful towards my ultimate goal.

My mindset in relation to the increased morning cardio sessions, has been to focus on the feeling of achievement that I get when I'm returning back to the house. I grab a cold drink, my clothes are wet with sweat (proof of my hard work), I have a wonderfully refreshing power shower, and I then can relax knowing that I already have the morning session in the bag. This is in comparison to getting up, putting the coffee machine on, starting work at the laptop within minutes, sitting back down, then starting a sedentary day of junk, sugar, ending with alcohol feeling stressed out and guilty.

The mindset improvement is working. I know deep down that I'll achieve my goals. Whether I'll achieve the weight loss target in the time period or not, I have no idea, but what I do know is that I'm not stopping.

My body is feeling different. It is difficult to really put into words except the movement of my body everyday has woken my body up. I feel different. I love the feeling of my heart, lungs, and blood pumping harder as I exercise. I do have to be careful considering that my resting heart rate was over 85 beats per minute. This is another reason that I've adopted a slow but consistent programme. I don't want a heart attack in the woods!

In other news, I am delighted to see another 2lb dropped this week. This isn't huge but it is consistent and moving in the right direction. Numbers can get a little meaningless so I always imagine a bag of sugar and then imagine one of them dropping from my body weight. 2lb doesn't sound a lot, but a bag of sugar is quite heavy.

Nutrition today has been:

- Granola and strawberries for breakfast.

- Duck poached eggs on sour bread toast for lunch.

- Thai green curry for dinner with beansprouts, mushrooms, brown rice and cashew nuts.

Exercise was the hike in the morning. I'm delighted to be now walking for over 60 minutes and I'm running that bit more every day. I'm tackling the hills with more gusto, and my need to stop, bend over, and fight for breath is lessening.

28 April 2020

I've made a huge decision today to stop drinking alcohol until my goal has been achieved, then I'll assess how I feel. As I do the cooking at home, I got into the habit of having a wine or two as I did it. This started off as 'me time' after a busy and often stressful working day. 'Me time' started to grow and as I cooked I would have my laptop on the kitchen island playing music, and I'd switch back and forth between answering messages, posting on social medial, and replying to emails. One or two wines became three or four wines and then the wine was replaced by gin. Up until today I would be knocking back over 2 litres of gin a week with no bother whatsoever. This has been a habit that I have enjoyed but is not good and has been pouring over 5000 calories a week into my body.

I did have a concern how I would feel at gin time. I'm pleased to say that I didn't miss it as much as I thought I would. I did my afternoon/evening session, had a shower, then cracked on and cooked the meal. I didn't mess around dragging out the cooking time due to enjoying drinking. I've broken the habit for the first time in a long time and it was totally fine.

I reckon that I've been burning around 5000 calories through hard work exercising. It's crazy to work so hard and then waste all that effort by consuming all that alcohol each evening. I'll never out train that. I don't expect the next few days to be as easy, but my health has to be my motivation.

Today's nutrition has been:

- A pint of spring water at 6am.
- Granola and strawberries for breakfast (after my morning session).
- Poached duck eggs on cheese on brown toast for lunch.
- Baked salmon in lemon and pepper, boiled new potatoes, mushrooms, and spinach in English mustard.
- I've drunk around 7 pints of spring water today.

I'm feeling really positive tonight. Stopping drinking has been a huge thing for me and I know that it is the right thing.

1 May 2020

Today was a huge day. I spoke to Pete this afternoon and we set the date for the National Three Peaks Challenge and we also agreed that we would go for this within 24 hours. Pete is going to fly up to Glasgow the night before and meet us. We shall have a lie in Tuesday morning, make the most of an easy day and then get to the foot of Ben Nevis for around 6pm. Amanda, who is our driver for the 24 hour challenge will wait in the car. By the time we climb to the top of the mountains dawn should look amazing, as long as the weather and visibility holds out for us.

We have also decided to raise money for charity. As we are all in the property business, and as Covid-19 is dreadfully affecting the homeless, we have decided to dedicate the challenge to Crisis who are a very worthy charity for homeless people. I've put the post out on Facebook and I'm blown away by the generosity of a £500 donation from Rob Hunter of Bond Housing Group. I'm truly moved by such an act of kindness.

So I have twelve weeks to prepare for the challenge. I'm going to have to step up my training for this. I not only have an obligation to myself to complete this, but I also have an obligation now to Pete, Amanda, and everyone who supports Crisis.

Today's nutrition was:

- A pint of spring water followed by two fresh coffees.

- Breakfast was granola and raisins.

- Lunch was a large poached goose egg, two rashers of bacon, and two granary toast.

- Dinner was king prawn, mushrooms, spinach, cashew nuts, pad Thai and basmati rice.

- I drank around six pints of spring water during the day.

Today's exercise was a 70 minute hike/run around the farm circuit and this afternoon I did 40 minutes on the rowing machine. I managed 6200m in that time. I'm struggling around 30 minutes with aching in my lower back so that last 10 minutes is getting pretty hard.

A big day today, I'm super revved up, but there is a lot of hard work to come.

2 May 2020

A shock to the body today as I packed a back pack with 2x 5kg weights for this morning's exercise. I've been struggling a little with a twinge in my right knee so I really didn't want to run and put more stress onto the joint and to be honest, I wouldn't have got far trying to run with this added weight.

This extra weight was a real test for the uphill slogs. I'm trying to put as much strength into my legs at the moment. I can't have my legs giving out on my during the Three Peaks. I kept the timings around 70 minutes but next week I need to increase this to around 80 minutes and possibly add another 5kg.

The kettlebell exercises are going well and I'm now starting to work harder on the core. This is positive move because a better core strength will help me with the climb in 12 weeks.

Nutrition was:

- My old favourite, Thai green curry. I'm loving eating well. I put the chicken in along with mushrooms, spinach, and cashew nuts for the fibre and good fats. Served with brown basmati rice and a few boiled new potatoes (my favourite) for varied texture.

I'm not sure whether this is a negative or a positive but this evening I craved a drink at the usual time. The feeling didn't last long. I thought, what's toughest, an hour long sweaty slog or simply resisting a few drinks?

Saving the best event of the day till last, I had my weigh in today and I'm down to 110.9kg from 113.7kg last week. A pretty big acceleration in weight loss which at the moment I believe has a lot to do with knocking the drink on the head. I'm happy.

4 May 2020

Gosh today was tough. My head wasn't in the right place at all so doing the two sessions was incredibly difficult. I'll never stop being amazed how much mindset totally affects one's ability to train and maintain a healthy lifestyle. At least that is the way it is for me. Today was the release of the full details on the Business Bounce Back Loans. This was totally in my mind during the morning session and gosh did I struggle to concentrate on doing my exercise.

As the hours went by, so did my frustration increase because our bank was not onboard with the scheme yet. By the time I got to session two (weights), I just wasn't in the mood anymore. However I forced myself to do it and whilst it was hard, I was proud to complete the session. This set me up for a relaxed evening knowing that I had completed what I had to complete.

Mindset is EVERYTHING.

I did introduce something new and positive today. I've started drinking fresh lemon water first thing in the morning. A friend recently suggested this to me and when I researched this it certainly seems as though there are some significant health benefits. I squeezed half a fresh lemon into around half a pint of spring water. It's not bad at all. Lemon helps boost metabolism for the day, and it's a great injection of vitamin C. Lemon cleanses the gut, and it also aids digestion. I've long suffered with indigestion so I'm hoping that with the elimination of the alcohol and the introduction of the lemon water I should start seeing some benefits.

Another reminder today of how I let myself slip, I was looking at BMI calculator today and when I put my numbers in I was told that I am 'slightly obese'. I really don't want to be obese.

Today's nutrition was:

- Lemon water.

- Granola and banana for breakfast.

- Poached eggs and cheese on toast.

- Salmon, new potatoes, mushrooms, two poached eggs, spinach and all washed down with a gallon of spring water.

Today's fitness was a one hour hike with 10kg on my back and then 50 minutes on the weights later in the day.

5 May 2020

So twelve weeks today Pete and I shall be starting our 24 hour Three Peaks Challenge. I'm now around 17.5 stone. I really need to get down to 15 stone. 14 stone being my final target on 31 August 2020. Over the next four weeks I'm going to maintain the same training as I am doing now. I'll then increase the level of training in small incremental steps.

I do however need to push the nutrition to the next level now. I'm a week on from cutting all the alcohol and apart from two or three moments, I haven't missed it at all. Neither have I missed putting 5000 calories into my body over the week.

I'm now going to focus on getting those testosterone levels up. Over the next four weeks I'm going to reduce my consumption of milk and cheese. Oestrogen is a female hormone that is found is cow's milk and cheese. I know that this won't be easy as I love milk in coffee and tea. I also really love quality cheese after a meal, but there seems little point in me concentrating on eating quality foods to support my testosterone levels and then reducing them back down by producing higher levels of oestrogen. Today I cut the coffee to just one cup. No cheese.

Amanda and I have also been thinking about becoming pescatarians. We aren't 100% on board with this yet but our weekly consumption is now around 60/40 in favour of fish over meat. Tonight I cooked a really nice stir fry with king prawns. We both love king prawns, salmon, tuna steak, scallops, mussels, squid, sea bass, trout, haddock, and cod. I really don't think that moving away from meat will be too difficult at all. As for the dairy products, we shall transition to alternatives by the end of the month and see how we get on.

So today's nutrition was:

- Lemon water first thing.

- Banana and granola for breakfast.

- Cheese on toast with poached eggs on top for lunch.

- King prawn in oyster sauce with brown basmati rice, mushrooms, cashews nuts, mushrooms and spinach.

- I drank are a gallon of spring water.

Today's exercise was the usual routine in the morning for an hour followed by 40 minutes on the rowing machine later in the day. I really struggled today. Applying for the Business Bounce Back Loans has been stressing me out so my head hasn't been fully into the exercise, but I still did it and I'm pleased that I did.

8 May 2020

I've been recommended the book '*The Obesity Code*' by Dr Jason Fung. I hate reading because it reminds me of study, so I usually buy audio books. Wow, I'm around 3 hours into the book and gosh it is good. I learned something new today that makes complete sense.

Over the last decade of gradually weight gain, I've experienced my fair share of stress. The Great Recession (2008), a redundancy, a nasty divorce, umpteen times in court dealing with child custody issues and then some more serious stuff that ended with Jack and Emma coming to live with us full time.

Then, the stresses of running four businesses, and more recently the Covid-19 pandemic. I've always put excess eating and excess drinking down to the need for comfort in times of stress, but I've never understood why. When we get stressed the stress hormone is released.

Cortisol is one of the main hormones released by the adrenal gland in response to stress. Basically, cortisol affects metabolism and how your body deposits fat. This can increase appetite, leading to weight gain, and in particular lead to extra deposits of fat in the abdomen. Our body assumes that stress may mean famine so it prepares for hard times by storing as much fat as it can whilst it reduces energy expenditure, by lowering our metabolism.

Over the past couple of days I have managed to keep the momentum going but the mindset hasn't been in a great place due to the stress of trying to get the businesses covered though obtaining the BBBLs. The mornings have been great, a new fresh day to wake up to, but the stress has built up in the afternoons and so I just haven't wanted to train. What I have done is to revert to a lesser session on the rowing machine. I can do a 30 minute session listening to some loud music as I try and switch off.

A weights session would be simply too hard whilst stressed. I have also had a twinge in the right knee which has made climbing very difficult. I'm still carrying the extra 10kg in my rucksack, but have chosen a more gentle cross country circuit. Over the past couple of days I have increased the morning session to 90 minutes which I'm very pleased about.

Today's nutrition has been:

- Lemon water first thing.

- Granola, and banana after morning session.

- Lunch was Eggs Benedict on wholemeal toast.

- For dinner I had salmon with new potatoes, mushrooms, spinach and a poached egg.

- I've drunk around a gallon of spring water today.

The big result of the day was 2.2lbs (1kg) less on the scales. I perhaps expected a little more off considering the elimination of alcohol, and the constant training, but this month so far, I am 9lbs lighter than three weeks ago, so that's a total of 13lb for the month. I'll take that!

9 May 2020

A BIG decision made

Today (tonight) starts the first day intermittent fasting. I'm going for 24 hour fasts every other day. The research that I've done for over 40s suggest that rather than 16:8 fasting every day, a more intense 24 hour fast every other day will be more beneficial.

I know that the time is right. I don't snack now, and I've cut the coffee (with milk and sugar) down. I'm not missing the alcohol, I'm not missing the sweet fizzy drinks, and I'm firmly into the fitness regime. Therefore, I see no point in delaying this huge step any further.

I have a goal for the Three Peaks so I shouldn't delay any more. I'm a little nervous to be honest because I don't want to find that fasting is really difficult for me and I have a huge setback with my mindset.

I'm also going to have to take some pressure off my right knee. Today my knee started hurting again as I did the morning hike. I can't afford to continue and risk making this a chronic injury. My knee has ached all day and I was in two minds whether I could even go on the rowing machine. So I reduced the resistance on the rower, and rowed for 34 minutes with no problems.

I'm going to lay off the impact exercise for a couple, or a few, days to let my knee recover.

Nutrition has been the usual:

- Lemon water, banana, strawberries granola, in the morning.

- Goose egg, bacon, cheese and mushroom omelette for lunch.

- King prawn Thai red curry for dinner.

- Around a gallon of spring water.

Exercise was a 92 minute hike this morning, and then a lighter 34 minute session on the rowing machine this afternoon.

A huge boost for me has been trying on my favourite jacket. Up until now I've not been able to fasten it. Today I tried it on and it fastens just great. I'm so happy.

10 May 2020

A tough day today!

I was absolutely fine with fasting until around noon. Up until that point I had been drinking a mix of straight ground coffee and several glasses of water. However from noon until 5.30pm it was extremely tough. I think today being a Sunday, and being on lockdown, has made matters worse as I had little to keep my mind occupied.

However, what was remarkable was the result on the rowing machine in the morning. As I am trying to let me knee rest I replaced the usual outside session with rowing. My previous personal best distance thus far has been 6.5km. Today I stopped at 10km and I could have gone further. I felt fantastic. I'm not sure whether it was a coincidence but rowing on an empty fasted stomach felt so much better than rowing several hours after eating lunch.

The afternoon's weight session felt different too. I maintained the same level of exercise but now understand from my research the benefits of exercising in a fasted state. After 20 hours growth hormones are released. These growth hormones can help me build muscle. Knowing this helps me get through the fast.

Nutrition for the day was very simple.

- Water and black coffee in the morning.

- Water and green tea in the afternoon.

- The fast was broken with a bowl of strawberries.

- Evening meal was fresh pan seared tuna, new potatoes,

green beans, and mushrooms cooking in English mustard.

I have mixed feelings on fasting having done my first day. I didn't enjoy it but I know that I'll have to get used to this. I'm going to start drinking more green tea in the afternoon as I understand that this can help with the feelings of hunger.

For now though, I'm going to do a 20:4 fast every other day. These will be the days that I do the weights in the afternoon so that I can make the most of the growth hormones that will be released towards the end of my fast. The decision to go every other day is based on two things:

i)   I understand that over 40s benefit from the variation of alternate day and,

ii) I just simply don't want to do a fast every day. I have to live with a regime that I can enjoy, doing this everyday will make me want to stop. This journey has to be sustainable.

11 May 2020

Not a great deal to report today considering I hurt my back yesterday doing weights.

A few years ago someone crashed into the rear of my stationary car whilst I sat in a traffic jam on the motorway. I could barely walk and ended up attending therapy sessions for over six months. Every now and again I get a twinge and it restricts my movement for a few days. This isn't a bad twinge today but enough to stop doing the heavier exercising for a few days. I'll go out for a walk later today, but it will be light stuff, no weights in my backpack.

Amanda and I went over to pick up our bikes from one of our properties. We haven't biked for years now so it's going to be fun to get back in the saddle as soon at my back is better.

Nutrition today (no fasting today) was:

- The usual lemon water, banana, and granola in the morning.

- A goose egg, cheese, bacon, and mushroom omelette for lunch.

- A power house dinner of sirloin steak, a piece of tuna, poached goose egg, mushrooms, spinach and cashew nuts sautéed in English mustard.

16 May 2020

7lb loss!

It has been a few days since my last diary note. The reason being that nothing new really happened over the past few days. I'm getting used to fasting and if I'm pleased to say that it's getting easier. Today's fast was just short of 23 hours and I could have gone longer if I needed to. I'm also starting to like the taste of green tea which really helps with the hunger waves in the afternoon.

The massive news of the day is that I weighed myself this morning. I actually weighed myself twice because I couldn't quite believe the scales. Over the past week I've dropped 7lbs! I can only put that acceleration down to the introduction of intermittent fasting. Whilst I'm getting used to the introduction of fasting I'm not increasing my exercise regime. The fasting must have been a big shock to the body so I don't want to over stress by increasing the exercise, and it doesn't look as though I need to. I'll see how it goes.

I'm very happy where I am in regards to what I am eating and drinking, I'm not planning on making any big changes there. Cutting out the processed food is complete. The introduction of the new whole food has been made. The best of all is that I can easily live with these choices. If I can live with these then I have every chance of keeping this up.

23 May 2020

5.2lb loss!

Another landmark day for me here. Another great week of weight loss with a 5.2lb loss. It is clear to me now, that the biggest accelerator in this whole process has been the introduction of intermittent fasting.

The exercise is great, cutting out alcohol is great, the whole food diet is great, dropping all the refined carbs is great. Drinking water is great, green tea is great, and lemon water is great, but over the past two months the huge success has come from the fasting.

It now makes so much sense that the fasting is the major driver in all this. In a 45 minute session on the rowing machine I'll burn around 350 calories. This is good because it gets the heart pumping, the blood flowing, the lungs pumping, and the muscles working, but as a pure weight loss tool how does that compare to fasting?

We know that an average man will burn around 2500 calories in a normal day. That is just the body functioning. This maintains Mr Average's current weight. A 45 minute session on a rowing machine is worth 350 calories, but it takes a deficit of 3500 calories to lose 1lb of fat. A calorie deficit of 500-1000 per day will help Mr Average lose 2lb a week. This is the theory but the theory is flawed. There isn't a calorie receipt in the brain, there isn't one anywhere in the body. Our body doesn't recognise one calorie from another (what's better? 200 calories of kale, or 200 calories of cake?)

If Mr Sports Drink gets on a rower and expends 350 calories - according to the rower - and Mr Water gets on the rower and also does 45 minutes, who will burn more fat?

It won't be Mr Sports Drink with his added glucose for energy. His insulin levels will be sky high so he will be burning the sugar in energy drink, or the other carbs he had through his energy bar earlier that morning.

Mr Water's insulin is low because Mr Water has been fasting (and he doesn't touch drinks with sugar or sweeteners), so the 350 calories will be taken from his fat stores.

We can now see why fasting outperforms diet, and why calorie counting is a pointless exercise.

I'm also more than delighted that Amanda has joined me with intermittent fasting. She is now on day 3 and is really embracing this. We are on different strategies. Amanda is doing 16:8 on a daily basis unlike my strategy of up to 22 hours every other day. We popped out for some shopping last night and she bought a box of turmeric tea and a box of ginger tea instead of the usual sweetened fizzy drink. I can't wait for her to start seeing, and more importantly, feeling the results. For me personally, I feel happy that my own actions and success have inspired her.

My bike came out today for the first time in years. I've been getting a little bored of the same routine so it's time to introduce something new. I took the bike down into the town and hit the canal path. The canal path is great. There are good stretches of level path but then those intermittent climbs around the locks, or over bridges, get those quick injections of anaerobic exercise. So 75 minutes for my first journey out which was respectable. My intention is to do a couple of bike rides each week gradually extending the distance and duration in small incremental steps. I must say though, my bum was numb, I'd forgotten that the seat is like a shard of rock! Amanda has ordered some padded cycling shorts for me.

Nutrition today was:

- The usual granola for breakfast with strawberries and banana.

- A mushroom, bacon, and cheese omelette for lunch.

- Smoked haddock with boiled baby new potatoes, poached egg, mushrooms, spinach, and cashew nuts (in English mustard) for dinner.

- Lemon water first thing followed by spring water during the day.

Exercise was the bike ride the morning and 35 minutes on the rowing machine at 5pm. I'm hoping that my back has settled down enough now to start some light weights again.

24 May 2020

Accountability

I want to mention the importance of sharing and accountability. Today I posted my month two accountability on Facebook. The post received 80 likes and 125 wonderful comments. It also attracted the most wonderful personal messages from people telling me how inspired they have been by seeing my return to health and fitness and how they have started their own campaign too.

I have to say, that the reaction from family, friends, and people I have never met has been a huge boost to my motivation to get this weight loss and fitness regime done. I don't care who you are, there will be days when the fasting feels more difficult than usual and you just want to break it to eat your favourite foods. There will be times when you just don't want to go out exercising at 7am, especially when the bed is lovely and warm and comfy. There will be times when demands from external sources are pulling on your attention, and so stopping work to go and lift weights just doesn't feel possible. To have the support of well-wishers, and to have the accountability that you set yourself has been priceless for me.

At some level we all need some form of support, recognition, and accountability from other people.

Today's nutrition was the fast until 5pm (from 7pm last night).

- A banana after the afternoon exercise session at 5pm.

- Dinner was at 7pm and was tuna steak, poached egg, small boiled new potatoes, mushrooms, spinach and cashew nuts in English mustard.

- During the fast I've drank plenty of spring water and green tea, and black coffee in the morning.

I missed out the morning exercise today. I felt as though I needed a break this morning as I felt too tired. It is very important to listen to your body. I was absolutely cool with missing this morning as I still had the afternoon session to do. As I fasted today I had the benefit of exercising in the fasted state to maximise the session.

Before I sign off for the night, I would strongly recommend that you find at least one person to be accountable to. This really does help.

28 May 2020

My Feet!

This is incredible. For the past few years, probably around 8 years, I have suffered with really sore feet. I have callouses around my heels and the balls of my foot, and they get so thick they crack leaving me with deep slits. They are incredibly painful. Emma says that the soles of my feet are made of stone, they are that hard. I've long put this down to living in houses without carpeting and being barefoot.

I looked into how you get callouses and read that this condition could be caused through vitamin deficiencies, namely vitamin C, vitamin B-3, and vitamin E. I didn't do much about it. I blamed the stone floors and the wooden floors.

Around a month ago I noticed that my feet weren't as bad as they usually are. As of now that healing has been continuing and the skin is getting softer. This is remarkable and demonstrated something fantastic to me. Healthy eating is crucial and if this is an outward show of lack of health, what the heck is happening on the inside?

As the chief cook and bottle washer, I'm also learning new and exciting dishes which I can make from scratch. Mine and Amanda's most favourite dish of all time is the Pakistani speciality Lamb Nihari. This is a thick meaty lamb stew/curry from the Indian subcontinent. It consists of slow-cooked meat, ideally lamb shank or beef, or mutton, goat or chicken, along with bone marrow. We first ate this at our favourite restaurant in Bradford, and it's delicious. This is a real treat after fasting, although a real tease because it is made from spices and herbs from all over the world, the smell of the cooking is a mouth-wateringly long 6 hours.

The other milestone is that last night / today I extended my fasting to 28 hours. Technically 28 hours but then I broke it with just a banana until I eat again after a further 2 hours. I exercised at around 27 hours to max out the benefits of the fast and those growth hormones, but being honest it was too much to exercise at that time. I was shattered and started to get cramping in the mid-section of my back. I had to finish a little early.

I found the fast quite easy though. The hunger waves come at the usual meal times but they soon go. When they came I drank black coffee, green tea or water. Amanda is doing great. She did an 18 hour fast today which is more than her usual 16:8.

In other news Emma, my daughter, is also eating healthier. This has been three weeks now. She also walks down to the local town to see her friends, now that she can, and back up the hill again. I haven't documented this as I wondered if it could be a fad for her, and she gives up. I don't think it is though and I'm delighted that this change in my life is rubbing off on another loved one.

Nutrition today was:

- Lamb Nihari this evening with brown basmati rice and cashew nuts.

- Plenty of water during the day as well as black coffee, green tea and ginger tea.

Exercise was a 70 minute hike with 10kg in the rucksack this morning, and a session on the rowing machine in the afternoon.

29 May 2020

2.8kg lost!

Following a 28 hour fast I would have thought the next 'off day' would have been a struggle to stop myself wanting to binge. It's strange though, I have no desire to over-eat whatsoever. I didn't want any breakfast today and so I just went straight through to lunch.

Lunch was just a goose egg omelette with mushrooms and cheese and nothing else. I'm now experiencing the difference between fasting and dieting. Apart from the huge differences in results, fasting isn't giving me any cravings or desire to binge on food. I simply feel comfortable with food not being a main focus in my life.

Amanda has also said something today that I can resonate with. She has significantly cut down on her desire to eat crisps, chocolate, and wash it all down with fizzy drink. This is a great place to be. She is now 'in the zone' and I fully expect her to constantly build on her achievements thus far.

The big news of the day for me is the weekly weigh in. I've hit 101.5kg. Another huge drop of 2.8kgs in the week. For the first time in years I'm in the 15 stone range. I'm feeling fantastic about this. At the rate I should be in the mid 14 stone range when I do the Three Peak Challenge which is ahead of schedule. The chance of achieving the challenge has just had a huge boost with this weight loss. The last thing I need is to to be heaving unwanted excess fat up 10,000ft if I don't have to.

Today was another mindset test. I'm dealing with a business issue that is causing me some significant stress. Stress increases my cortisol levels, and that is when I often lose the motivation to exercise, so I really need to accept that I'll deal with what I can. Then I'll put it in a box until the next time it needs to be dealt with. That way the matter is dealt with, as much as I can at the moment, without the usual unnecessary nagging stress that I always allow myself to suffer from.

I thought that I would document what is happening with the exercising regime of late. I still aim to exercise twice daily but there has been the occasional day when I've missed a morning or afternoon session. This is only because I've listening to my body and it's told me 'No, not now. You aren't doing this, Fernley'. I haven't increased intensity or duration over the past three or four weeks. I'll share my reasons for this

i)   Because I'm still trying to protect my right knee and lower back from increased stress. Running isn't right for me at the moment. Starting out, impacting these almost 50 year old joints with 19 stone of body weight isn't a particularly good idea. Even as my weight drops down to 18st, 17st, and 16st there is still a lot of weight on my joints. I've found that replacing the run with a fast hike with the additional

10kg in the back pack a much kinder experience on the body, and for that matter actually a much more enjoyable experience for me. If you are going to exercise on a daily basis then it is crucial that you find something you enjoy. If you dread your session it won't last because you'll find any excuse to give up.

ii)   My current focus is on losing the excess weight. There seems little point in trying to build muscle if it is lost under a layer of fat. My concentration is on consistent aer-obic exercise to keep my body moving, and burning that unwanted body fat. The last thing I need to do is cause stress to my body, which increases the stress hormone, cor-tisol. Cortisol causes fat storage. Dreading the sessions, and seeing little happen with the fat loss, and getting totally demotivated, is not a good tactic.

My current exercise regime is all based around enjoyable, con-sistent, aerobic sessions. I shall need to step this up for the Three Peaks Challenge but at the moment I'm focused on drop-ping the fat. Dragging unnecessary fat up the mountains is the last thing I will need. Neither am I concentrating on weights. My back still doesn't feel great so I've cut the weights to just my arms and shoulders until my back feels strong enough to take the strain.

4 June 2020

Scafell Pike

The day has arrived. Today I would climb the 3281ft, 6 miles, 5 hours up Scafell Pike, the highest mountain in England with Pete, his sister Bee, and my son Jack.

This was going to be a test for the big National Three Peak Chal-lenge in seven weeks. I have worked hard up until this point but this was going to be the test. When I made a commitment to get back to fitness on 26 March 2020 there would be no way that I could have undertaken this climb. I was too fat, carrying far too much weight, with weak muscles, and no stamina. I remember my first day training and going for a morning walk to find myself bent over gasping for air as I climbed the valley at the bottom of our fields. What I was to do today was probably 100 times harder than that short climb.

Leading up to today I have done two back-to-back 23 hours fasts as my fast day coincided with the climb. There was no way that I was going to fast and undertake this hike on the same day. I prepared the day's food for myself and Jack. I packed a number of cheese and ham sandwiches, fruit, and 4 litres of spring water. It would be important to feed regular energy coming into my body whilst also staying hydrated.

I was a little nervous before the climb as I'd never climbed a mountain before, and certainly not coming from a place of such poor fitness and health. However, I am delighted to report that the climb went really well and we reached the summit in 2.5 hours.

It is a tough climb. The terrain is extremely rocky under foot which stresses the ankles, knees and every muscle. The climb is steep, and coming down really jolts the joints and tests the thigh muscles. There were three occasions when I couldn't keep up with Pete's pace but I kept pushing. The temperature difference at the car park is vastly different to the summit. As we were setting off, a chap was finishing his climb. "It's cold and windy up there" he said. "-3C" he stated. He was correct. I started the climb in a short sleeved T shirt. By the time I had reached the peak, I had a jumper and a jacket on and I was still freezing cold.

We finished the hike in 5 hours and 30 minutes. It was a respectable time as we had taken the longer more scenic route down, back to the car park. Sitting in a comfy car seat was like heaven.

Today was a huge milestone for this journey back to health. I'm shattered but I feel on top of the world. The next challenge is to the Yorkshire Three Peaks.

5 June 2020

100kg!

Not a great deal different to report today except that the weigh in is 100kg! That is over 3lbs for the week. It's decent but not on the scale of the past 3 to 4 weeks which have been huge. I may be getting to a levelling off period for a while until I step this up again. Plateaus are great on mountain climbs, but not with weight loss.

To hit my 5 stone goal by the end of August, I have 11kg to lose in just 12 weeks. This should be easily achievable though. I'll need to keep pushing on the fitness, start pushing again on more resistance, and push harder on more climbs. The intermittent fasting continues as does the nutrition regime.

11 June 2020

Wales is still in Lockdown

Other news is that it's looking unlikely that Wales is going to open up its Lockdown so we can't travel to Snowdon for a while yet. Clearly this is a major issue considering that Snowdon is one of the three mountains on the challenge.

Pete sent me through an alternative to the Three Peaks and I'm loving the challenge of this one. The Cairngorms 4000s is a climb up the five mountains, that all over 4000 feet, in the Cairngorms National Park within 24 hours. The mountains are:

- Cairn Gorm (1245m)
- Ben Macdui (1309m)
- Cairn Toul (1291m)
- Sgnor and Lochan Uaine (1258m)

- Braeriach (1296m)

Noting that Snowdon is 1085m and Scafell Pike is 978m, this will be a huge step up in physical assertion. Of course I've accepted the challenge, although I'll be honest, it fills me with the fear of failure.

The Yorkshire Three Peaks

Pete and I have also decided to slot the Yorkshire Three Peaks in next Friday and I cannot wait. This is going to prove to be a significant test over and above that of Scafell Pike last week. Whilst none of the Yorkshire peaks are as high as Scafell Pike, the route is 24 miles, includes a climb of 1585m, and needs to be completed with 12 hours. As I write this, I still can't believe that my body is able to take these challenges on after I've neglected it so badly.

Diploma in Nutrition

In other news I've completed my first Diploma in Nutrition. There were 16 modules and 8 have already been assessed. I'm delighted to say that I've achieved a Distinction in all 8 units. I'll take a couple of days off now before cracking on with the Advanced Diploma.

Possibly the biggest news to report is mine and Amanda's intention to start cutting meat and dairy from our diet. As someone who loves eating quality meat, and isn't that keen on many plant based foods, this is going to prove to be a test. However, I've been researching the potential negative effects on the body through meat consumption, and in particular processed meat, along with dairy and dairy based foods.

We are going to start experimenting with a plant based diet. Whether that will ever go to full on Vegan, or stick around as Flexitarian diet, I'm not sure at this time, but for now sausages, bacon, ham, tinned tuna, and bratwurst are going to be used up and not replaced. I've little to no experience in cooking plant based meals so I need to do some research and experimentation as processed vegan food is as bad as any other processed food.

Today's nutrition was:

- Early morning lemon water.
- Banana and granola for breakfast.
- Mushroom soup and toasted sourdough bread for lunch.
- King prawns with mushrooms, spinach, cashew nuts in chow mein sauce on a bed of brown rice.
- A gallon of spring water throughout the day.

Fitness was a steady 70 minutes hike this morning with 40 minutes on the rowing machine.

12 June 2020

1.5kg lost!

Just a quick update as it's Friday and that means its weigh-in day. I'm very pleased to record another consistent drop of 1.5kg which takes me down to 98.5kg. I'm on the home straight now to achieve the target goal.

The huge losses now seem to have ceased which is only to be expected as I get closer to my optimal weight.

14 June 2020

Trying out vegan for size

Armed with a trolley full of shopping from the vegan shopping expedition last night, it was time to try our first vegan dish.

Macaroni cheese was on the menu but with organic spinach pasta. We have never tried vegan cheese before so this was a new one for us, along with almond milk, garlic, and other usual ingredients. The result had mixed feedback. Emma loved it and wanted more. Jack said that he enjoyed it. I thought it was bland with little texture or taste, and I doubt Amanda will be ever having it again.

Amanda's feedback may be a little tough on the mac and cheese itself because she has never been a pasta fan. Part way through the meal Amanda and I resorted to cutting four pieces of sour bread and putting them into the toaster. The toast at least gave the dish some more flavour and texture. The butter wasn't vegan.

Other feedback was that chocolate flavoured almond milk is a huge hit with Emma, now a trainee vegan I think. The vegan cheese tasted okay and might be a reasonable substitute in such servings as melted cheese on toasted sour bread. Amanda has found a vegan organic yogurt and the feedback was that it was a winner.

Clearly today is too early to decide on how many animal based foods will be replaced by plant based foods, but we now realise that over the next few weeks we shall undergo a trial and error exploration into vegan foods.

Whilst of course not set in stone, our intentions shall be able to cut down on a number of animal based products where we can. We can replace a lot with enjoyable alternatives, and any meat and fish we'll restrict to line caught or grass fed where we can. Our intention is to at least eliminate processed meats i.e deli type meats, bacon, burgers, and sausages.

I've also revised my training regime. The focus so far has been on weight loss and so I've been pushing on the cardio aerobic sessions. This has been mainly hiking (with added weights) and rowing with some upper body weights. As I'm ahead of pro-gramme on the weight loss, and still losing, I'm switching back to a dedicated weights session every other day. The shops open tomorrow having been in lockdown since March and so I'd like to get over to the local town and see what additional weights I can pick up.

Another share of the day is a book that I'm currently listening to called '*10% Happier*' by Dan Harris. Early morning hiking on the moors is a great opportunity to put the audio books on and continue learning. The book was recommended to me by my friend Pete. It's gearing up to be a cracker and I look forward to sharing further on in this book.

19 June 2020

2.1kg loss

It was weigh-in day again and I'm delighted to log a 2.1kg loss for the week. The scales are now reporting 96.4kg and that 88kg goal is coming ever closer. Unless something totally unforeseen happens then I should be hitting the 5 stone loss in 4 months.

It's my 50th birthday in eight days. It would be an amazing birthday present to be in the 14's (stone) when I turn 50. All I have to do is carry on with the current regime and there should be no reason for not hitting that weight.

We were due to go to Ingleborough today to tackle the Yorkshire Three Peaks Challenge but Pete asked if we could delay a week as he has a small injury following a heavy high intensity workout. 24.5 miles up and down hills wouldn't be any fun for him nursing an injury. We have scheduled for next Friday. The weather looks better than today at least. I really cannot wait. I haven't tackled a hike this distance before so hitting this a day before my 50th will be yet another birthday present to savour.

Mindset interrupted

I didn't record yesterday but I ought to record now what happened. I've written a lot about mindset and the importance of having the head in the right place to undertake a transformation. Yesterday was one of those days that is ever so difficult. Emma was in school that morning. The first school run since schools closed for lockdown. She had asked me if we could set off around 8.10am. This was right in the middle of my usual morning session that I had routinely built into my life for the past three months. Of course I agreed but I would get up earlier and get a 45 minutes session on the rower before I dropped her off, which would win me some time back.

I was woken by my alarm. Oh heck, Emma, school, time, rowing machine, time, but I'm tired, shall I do it later? I got up, totally at odds with myself and poured myself a glass of water. If I went on the rowing machine now then I could get 30 minutes in, I thought, but I was tired, felt rushed, and the last thing I wanted was to sit down on that machine.

I didn't exercise in the end, I just got myself ready and took Emma to school. The school run is around 30 minutes. When I got back I had a couple of messages and emails waiting for an answer. Then by the time I had answered those, a business based discussion had commenced with Amanda. It was now mid-morning and I was feeling guilty for not doing my planned morning exercise. Today was a fast day and for some reason, probably because my head wasn't in the right place the hours seemed to be going incredibly slowly and I was feeling wave after wave of hunger.

A letter arrived in the post for Amanda. It was concerning the service charges on an apartment she owns. The account had been put in dispute following a formal complaint made by us. The dispute wasn't replied to by the management company, and now they were trying to levy ridiculous late payment charges onto her bill. This arriving on our doorstep completely diverted my attention away from my exercise.

The afternoon was dominated by discussing this letter and how we would best deal with the problem. It was now 4pm and afternoon session time. I just didn't want to do anything. My head was filled with stress. I was suffering hunger waves and my head was translating them as bad rather than as good. Nothing

I had planned for the day had been completed, and I was supposed to switch off and exercise. I just didn't want to but I knew that if I didn't then all evening I would sit and wallow in remorse and guilt. That was worse than not making myself just do the exercise.

The hell with it! I went on the machine and endured a 30 minutes session which is an absolute minimum workout. I finished the session, which I hated, and then went into the kitchen to break the fast with a banana. As I went to shower, for the first time that day, I felt positive and back in control. What had happened that day? Surely there were lessons to be learned?

My routine had been broken, not by planning, but by events not aligning themselves with the time available. I'd endured feeling guilty all day rather than getting home from the school run, turning the phone off and then shutting the computer down for 30 - 45 minutes. I'd allowed the letter to dominate my thoughts and rather than deal with it, or shelve it for a more appropriate time. It got into my head which had allowed me to wreck the list of activities I had prepared early that day. During all that, I had craved food and started to resent the fast I had committed to. This is how I used to live. This is how I put so much weight on in the first place! This is why my blood pressure and heart rate had risen so much, and this is why I had struggled with mindset and then patched it up with alcohol.

20 June 2020

So, back to today. One of the great things about a night's sleep is that it always brings a new day. Today I awoke at 6am without the need for an alarm. I got up, drank the usual glass of water, checked social media, answered a couple of questions, made a list for the day, let the birds, dog, and goat out, and collected some freshly laid eggs. Got chased by our gander who is a complete pain in the arse during egg laying season, then got ready and went on the morning hike. Totally relaxed. Totally focused.

I got back around 8.30am and started producing content for the property coaching business. The house was still nice and quiet. The coffee machine was on, and I felt like a different man from the day before. The past two days has reinforced everything I have witnessed and learned about mindset.

So today was a no meat day for Amanda and I. I skipped breakfast because I simply wasn't hungry. Amanda was fasting until 1pm anyway.

- Lunch was omelette, Vegan cheese, mushrooms and spinach.

- Dinner was a pretty large serving of garlic mushrooms on sourdough bread. The garlic mushrooms are a big hit here. They are so tasty and rammed with superfoods. When I cook garlic mushrooms I cook in virgin olive oil, fresh garlic, and throw in fresh parsley. The nutrients in that dish are abundant.

- I consumed the usual lemon water, spring water, along with a couple of green teas.

Exercise was the hike this morning followed by a 40 minute weights session this afternoon.

21 June 2020

4 stone lighter

Today was the start of a shift in my focus on exercise. I've now lost a total of 4 stone, which I'm super thrilled about, with just one last stone to go. I expect to be around the 14 stone mark by the end of July which will have smashed my original goal of 5 stone in 5 months to bits. 5 stone in 4 months is a possibility! However, I need to start switching the aerobic exercise to more resistance work. I don't feel strong and fast enough and that needs to change.

So today I increased my back pack load by 50% to 15kg. This was quite a shock to the body but afterwards I felt great. I'm also focussing now on my core strength. My core is quite weak and not conditioned. I started off with four simple core exercises. Crunches, leg raises, plank, and then press ups. I found this really difficult but that's good. Lots to work on!

In other news I've found another challenge to have a go at. On the British Rowing website you can sign up to take part in virtual rows across various seas, oceans, and rivers. I've enrolled for the English Channel row which is 39,806m. The longest row I've done so far is 10,000 so this is a huge undertaking if I'm going to do it in the day (which I intend to do). I'll get the Yorkshire Three Peaks polished off this week and then aim to crack on with the row next week.

I've fasted today so not much of an update on the nutrition side.

- I did King Prawns in lemon, garlic, and black pepper which tasted wonderful. I make this from scratch, and the details are in the nutritional part of the book. Lots of water today.

Exercise was the usual hike this morning, but with the increased weight. This afternoon was resistance and core workout (really tough).

25 June 2020

The Yorkshire Three Peaks Challenge

Wow what a day that was. As I lay here, in bed writing this log, I can hardly move. Today was the Yorkshire Three Peaks 12 hour challenge and I have to say that I completely underestimated how tough the day would be. The three peaks are:

- Pen-y-Ghent (694 metres)
- Whernside (736 metres)

- Ingleborough (723 metres)

The weather was a scorcher at 30°C which made the challenge all the harder. I really should have appreciated how hiking almost the distance of a marathon, carrying up to 6 litres of water, over rocky and tough terrain, and ascending and descending the height of Ben Nevis, would be extremely tough.

Jack and I met with Pete and Bee bang on 5am. It was Pete's suggestion to meet at that time considering the weather was forecasting a heatwave. The first peak, Pen-y-Ghent, is only around 90 minutes and we had reached the summit by around 6.30am. On the way down Bee fell and hurt her knee. Sadly she had to pull out and head off back to the car.

I started to hurt when approaching the second peak which would have been around 50% of the total distance. The walk up to Whernside was long, not as steep as Pen-y-Ghent but really really long. By now the heat was really affecting us so the slog between Whernside and Ingleborough was tough. The hike felt never ending with this last peak bearing down on us. Approaching Ingleborough you can see some of the route up the side. It's that steep, it zig zags. Marvellous.

The climb up to Ingleborough is a messy clamber over really rocky terrain. I've never been so exhausted in my life. It was sheer hell. Pete had gone ahead (the guy is a machine) which left me and Jack trying to drag ourselves up to the summit. We eventually reached the top of the zig zag trail. I looked up and saw the next leg of steep uphill climb bearing down on us. My heart just sank. I honestly just fell to my hands and knees and felt like crying. 20 miles of heavy hike on tired legs and a load more climbing to do.

Jack and I reached the summit where Pete was waiting for us. The aim was to finish within 12 hours, but we had lost a lot of time climbing up Ingleborough so the timing was looking tight. From the summit to the car was around 4 miles and we had 1.45

hours to do it in. Heading back to the car was hard. My body was aching like crazy. I'd struggled with a sore muscle in my back. My poor thighs had been chafing for hours and we had run out of water. I was also getting waves of sickness which I guess was a consequence of the sun with fatigue. We knew that we had to maintain a decent pace now to beat the 12 hours.

I used the Strava app on my phone to monitor our pace. This was a great help because it's so easy when one's exhausted to slow down without realising. We arrived at the village, crossed the railway line, turned right over the bridge, and up what seemed like a never ending road to the car where Bee was waiting with ice cold drinks.

Challenge achieved in 11 hours and 53 minutes. Did it!

That was incredibly tough but gave me an appreciation of how far I had come with this fitness training but also how far I had to go. There is no doubt that The Yorkshire Three Peaks is a huge challenge but for the National Three Peaks I simply don't want to go through the same pain I went through today. It seems that both challenges are of a similar toughness. The Yorkshire perhaps being the tougher physically but the National is partly done in the dark and over a 24 hour period.

I know that I'll need to get a few more, longer climbs in between now and the National Three Peaks so as not to slow Pete down, complete the challenge within the 24 hours, and not go through what I went through today.

Tonight was a treat night so I popped into the shop for an ice cold lager and picked up some spicy lamb chops from the local take out.

I have to say that I'm incredibly proud that Jack came along with us. He hasn't trained at all for this but at 18 years old and with the physique of a marathon runner he got around without complaining or whining.

So, before I wrap up. That was a day I'll never forget. Experiences like this are simply not possible if you don't keep yourself fit and healthy. I'm so grateful.

Oh, and when I unpacked my rucksack I found 2 litres of water right at the bottom...!

26 June 2020

50 today!

My word where did half a century go? My body is aching today. There isn't much to record except that I've decided to enter the Manchester Marathon on 11 October 2020. This gives me 15 weeks to train, which gives me a fighting chance of success.

I want to do this because I want to see what can be achieved after so much obesity and inactivity. Perhaps more than that, I want to prove something to myself having turned 50. This might even be my second mid-life crisis.

I managed to get 40 minutes in on the rowing machine this afternoon which was surprising considering the amount of aching yesterday. The pain in my back muscle actually stopped me though due to the intensity of the feeling of muscle-burn.

Nutrition today was:

- Garlic mushrooms on toasted sour bread for lunch.
- Lamb Nihari and brown rice for dinner.

A birthday treat of 3 glasses of red wine was the order of the day. Spending so much less on alcohol means when I do have a treat, I can spend a bit more than usual and have a nicer, smoother wine.

29 June 2020

I've had to give myself a talking to this morning. Monday morning, raining outside and blowing a gale like it's a wet November day.

My head started thinking (stressing) about the VAT return, getting an apartment ready for letting, and many more things I didn't have to consider yesterday.

So, as per my regime, I set about my morning session on the rowing machine, but I really didn't want to. My legs are still aching from the Yorkshire Three Peaks and it's pouring down out there so no running or hiking this morning. This was one of the totally unmotivated, difficult, seemingly never-ending exercise sessions that we endure from time to time. I cut it off at 30 minutes and had a shower feeling a little fed up.

I've committed now to the marathon and we have the National Three Peaks in four weeks. I need to get cracking and get some increased endurance in the bag now. After the session, I connected with Pete who remains a massive support. He's a great help for getting the head aligned again. As a result of getting my head back in place, I've set a plan out for the week incorporating some increased leg work. Having a plan in place, and having completed the exercise, I was then able to crack on and focus on the business day ahead.

For this reason, I thought it might be a good idea to create a 'Monday Motivation' each Monday to support each other in the Facebook support group. Transformation can be lonely and easily given up. We all need support.

So I'll kick off with my motivation for the week ahead.

    1. Today, Wednesday, Friday, Sunday are 22 hour fast

days.

2. I want to hit 14 stone 7lb on weigh day Friday.

3. Continue the usual exercise regime but include 2 x 3 hours climbs (for 3 peak training)

4. Start running again this evening before dinner.

Having got over my morning wobbles I'm pleased to say that the fasting went well. It was in fact good to get back to fasting having had a few days out of routine due to the Yorkshire Three Peaks, my 50th, and the eating at irregular times.

Another huge mistake that I made this morning was doing something that I know not to do. I weighed myself only three days after the last weigh in. The double mistake was to weigh myself at a different time in the day. The result was that the scales told me that I have put on 0.5kgs since Friday. Clearly that isn't a reflection on fat gain but seeing that number rise, despite knowing that I shouldn't have weighed myself, did make me feel a little down and deflated. If you are reading this, for goodness sake don't be drawn into the lure of the scales. Weighing yourself too regularly can be bad for your mindset and motivation because your weight can naturally fluctuate.

Nutrition has been good today (another reason to be positive):

· I fasted until 5pm when I had my usual banana after the second exercise session.

· At 7pm I enjoyed pan fried cod loin in black pepper and fresh lemon, boiled new potatoes, asparagus, mushrooms and spinach in English mustard.

- Plenty of water, with fresh black coffee in the morning and a couple of green teas in the afternoon.

Running has to start slowly for me. As I twinged the knee a few weeks ago I have to be careful, so I opted for a 45 minute session of circuits around our fields. I ran on the level and downhill, whilst walking fast up the inclines. At the end of each circuit I grab the sledge hammer and pound 50 swings into a huge tyre before starting the next circuit. This really got the heart racing and was a great start to the marathon training.

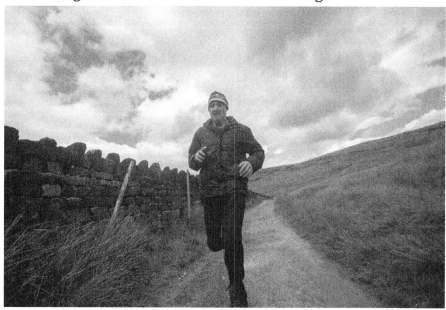

Running during a hike

3 July 2020

Weight loss plateau

I haven't journalled for a few days as there hasn't really been anything new to note. It's weekly weigh day and I'm wondering if I've hit the weight-loss plateau? I've only dropped 0.5 kilos for the week which has been the lowest weekly drop since I started. I know that this is to be expected at some point. I discuss this later in the book as there are umpteen reasons that people hit the weight loss plateau. The absolute important thing is not to get disheartened, understand that this happens, evaluate what is happening, adjust if necessary and carry on.

Whilst I'm not totally sure why the weekly drop has been so little, I can think a number of contributing factors that I would suggest haven't helped.

1. I know that I haven't been drinking as much water as I have been. It's easy to drift away from routine and not drinking enough water isn't good.

2. I drank some (not a great deal) of alcohol for three evenings at because it was my birthday this week.

3. Meal timings haven't been great and so fasting hasn't been as strict as it has been.

4. I was wrecked after the Yorkshire Three Peaks and so last Friday and Saturday were only very light exercise days due to my body aching.

5. I've noticed that I'm letting the carbs creep back into my diet. For 2 out of 3 days this week I've had cheese toasties. The kids got the sandwich toaster out and I couldn't resist.

After three months, it's just too easy to let these bad habits slip back into my life. Perhaps one or two slips wouldn't be noticed but five will.

I'm really pleased to note that the running is going well. Sadly we have had a week of rain here which isn't great, but I'm getting daily runs in and I'm still enjoying it.

Clothes shopping!

The most gratifying events over the past couple of days have been going shopping for new clothes now that shops are open after Lockdown. Being able to go and buy clothes that I actually like, rather than searching through the XXXL end of rail stuff has been bloody fantastic. I've bought a pair of 34" waist jeans for the first time in 10 years. I was a 40" waist. I'm also in size L shirts and T-shirts now rather than XXXL. This feels amazing.

I've been fasting today so nutrition has been:

· Black coffee in the morning with plenty of water.

· Dinner was Mediterranean Chicken and Roasted Vegetables.

· Green teas in the afternoon with water again.

Exercise of the day was a 40 minute row this morning followed by a 62 minute run. Whilst it was pouring down, it was exhilarating to be running in the elements. Nobody was out, it was just me.

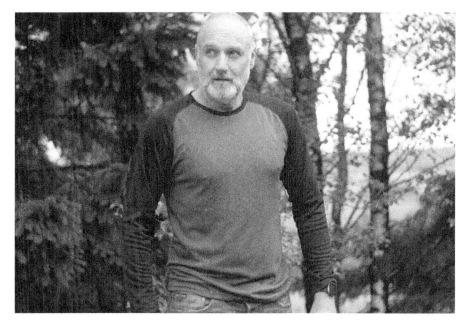

Man at C&A

6 July 2020

Snowdon

A last minute decision to head across to Snowdon with Pete today. We're now counting down to the National Three Peaks so we need to get some more mileage in the bag and test the timings. I'm delighted to say that the stamina is vastly improving as we managed to get up the Pyg track and down the Miners track in a respectable 3 hours and 22 minutes. It's a good slog up there but I'm seeing a huge difference in my leg strength and my recovery rate from that of a few weeks ago when climbing Scafell Pike.

I have to say though, that doing this sort of thing, climbing mountains and viewing world class mountain ranges with great company, would never have been possible in the state I was in. The whole exercise of figuring out and researching the route, setting a date, driving through beautiful countryside, parking up, looking up at a mountain, then climbing up it is just the best. Breathing in the freshest of air, experiencing the feeling of freedom, reaching the summit, and looking out across dozens of mountains toward the coastline is something money can't buy. I feel so grateful.

So a great day of activity under the belt, and whilst I don't count calories, the watch told me that I'd burned over 4500 calories for the day. I only mention the calories as an indication of my energy expenditure for the day.

In other good news, I've now hit the 14 stone 7lbs mark. After the short-lived weight loss plateau last week I've addressed the observations, adjusted, and have now continued the weight loss. Phew!

Today's nutrition was:

- A pack-up of sandwiches in granary brown bread

- Loads of lemon water.
- Dinner was a rib eye steak with poached eggs, and mushrooms in English mustard.

A rare treat, a lovely Zinfandel. I'd worked hard today.

Finally, I have discussed the importance of support and accountability and have noted the wonderful messages received over the past few weeks. Tonight was no exception. One of Jack's friends (18 years old) messaged me to ask if he could come along on one of our next challenges. Yes of course, was my reply. It's ever so fulfilling that this journey has reached out to people a generation younger than myself. This sort of thing means the world.

10 July 2020

A good positive day for weigh-in day. I've now broken into the 91 kilos range (just) at 91.9 kilos. The weight loss has certainly slowed down now but that is to be expected. I want to hit the 5 stone loss in 4 months which gives me just over a couple of weeks to achieve that goal. Considering the slow-down, I'm confident, but it will be tight.

Starting to run

This morning was the first day running on tarmac. The route would be from the farm, up over a short stretch of moorland, onto the road, then uphill for around 2 miles. Then down and back to the farm. This is a 4.6 mile circuit. The run went okay but quite slow. I completed the circuit in 59 minutes. The reason for the slowness is that I'm just not fit enough to run up hills. I've no chance. So using the steady but consistent strategy, I ran on the flat and the downhill, and walked the hills. Tomorrow I'll push a little harder, the day after a bit more, and so on. Weight trainers call this Progressive Overload.

If the marathon goes ahead then I'm under no illusion that to finish in a decent time the training will need to be significantly stepped up. There is a little over 13 weeks to go. Still being in fat loss mode, I'm not concentrating on the correct diet for endurance and strength training. I really need to get down to the goal over the next couple of weeks, get the National Three Peaks polished off, and start pushing hard on the fitness.

Chatting with Pete today, he thought if Manchester postpone the marathon due to social distancing then it could be a blessing in disguise which would give me another six months to put together a longer training period. I get that, but I want to push this and competing a marathon in as little as six months from being unable to walk up a hill without stopping for breath would be an incredible personal achievement.

With the increase in training now required, this afternoon's session was a mix of strength and cardio. Sledgehammer exercising, large tyre flips, and running. If I'm honest, I didn't enjoy it.

No fasting today so:

- Lemon water first thing.

- Banana and melon with loads of water until lunch.

- Garlic mushrooms, toasted sour bread, parsley and sage for lunch.

- Water and Green Tea leading up to dinner.

- A Lamb Nihari treat for dinner, then, into fast again.

11 July 2020

Only a very quick journal note today to record an improvement on the tarmac run this morning. Down from 59 minutes 1 second to 57 minutes and 23 seconds.

I'm recording this, not because I've knocked a minute and a half off my time, but because the improvement has made my day. The day started off with positivity, improvement and progress. Such a great way to start a Saturday.

A fasting day today. Two sessions. One run, weights and core.

There will have been a good percentage of fat burned off. Happy!

13 July 2020

I wanted to document today because I've let negative nonsense, from negative and nonsense people, out rank my health and fitness on my own priority scale. Never again will I allow this to happen. In business we get disputes, it's par for the course. What is also par for the course is to get stupid solicitor letters that need dealing with. We had one this afternoon. I'll not go into this, as it's very minor, but nonetheless a drain on time and energy if allowed. I let this dominate my afternoon, drag my mood down, ditch the fast, and scrap my afternoon session. Stupid!

Is this what we do? Do we allow distraction to damage our health? Yes. At least I am guilty of this and it needs to stop. It needs to stop now. It's crazy when we consider that we allow this negativity to throw us off so easily. Today has highlighted why I had so many false starts trying to gain my health back. I allowed stresses to dominate my life.

15 July 2020

Sadly the Manchester Marathon has been called off until April 2021. I must admit that I'm really disappointed as picking up a medal for such an achievement would have been hugely personally satisfying only six months after putting my walking boots on.

A couple of friends have suggested that I train anyway for running the distance on the day and record the achievement. It's a good idea. I'm still intending training for the marathon, but I'm considering what other challenges could I go for this year.

The National Three Peaks is still on though and as such today I've had two good sessions. This morning was a run, and this afternoon was a hike with a 15kg back pack

I've decided that I'm going to aim for five runs each week. I'm conscious that my knees and joints are 50 years old and to start pounding tarmac now, could lead to some trouble. A couple of days off running will give my legs chance to recover.

I can report a steady improvement on the past five days of running in terms of speed and distance. I believe that the increases, so early on, are due to:

i)   the body starts to get used to different activity and stresses very quickly, but more importantly

ii)   the 'The Roger Bannister Effect' or otherwise called the Psychological Breakthrough.

Nobody thought that it was possible to run 4 miles in under one minute. Runners tried and failed until a man called Roger Bannister crushed the 4 minute mile mark. What this did was show other runners that running a mile in under 4 minutes was achievable. As soon as they believed that a human being was able to achieve this, no longer held back by this psychological barrier, swarms of runners ran a mile also under 4 minutes.

In my own way, this has been the same principle for me. Day 1, I ran and struggled up the hills. Day 2, was that bit further, and that bit faster. Every day, I pushed a little more up the hill, a little faster down that hill, and the time comes down. So much comes down to belief.

A big fast day today, 24 hours. No problems at all. It's just a matter of getting used to it, knowing the hunger waves come, knowing how to deal with them, and knowing that food time is never that far away.

I have to note at this point, because it's come to mind having been walking around the shops this evening, that one of the other benefits of Intermittent Fasting is cost. The monthly food bill has been cut from around £900 to £500. It's huge. £4.8k per year. A whole food diet has seen the elimination of sweetened drinks, chocolate, cake, crisps, and of course the booze. I love getting fit and saving money as I go.

Today's nutrition has been:

- water, black coffees and afternoon green tea

- followed by chicken Thai red curry and brown rice for dinner.

Today's exercise has been the morning run, now at five miles, followed by a hike with weights in the evening.

19 July 2020

I have to journal today out of pure appreciation. This morning felt so special. It's been a rubbish June and July for weather, but this morning was glorious. A glorious Sunday morning. Up at 6.30am, took the dog out, a quick lemon water, a stretch of the legs, and then out into the country roads. The feeling of freedom in getting out and running is just the best. Now that the fitness is improving and I can start enjoying what I am doing means the experience is way beyond that of just getting fit. There is something more meaningful.

I'm a shade off 10km now at 9.7km. I'm taking my son Jack and his friend Alex to Helvellyn tomorrow for a great day's hiking. On Tuesday morning I'm going to crack the 10km run and I can't wait.

I'm also thinking that now is the time to ease back on the intermittent fasting from every other day, to 2x 24 hour fasts per week. I'm very close to my 70lb fat loss goal and starting to push harder into the strength and endurance. As such, I believe the time has come to start concentrating on nutrition to help with the demands that I intend to place on the body. I'm not sure as yet if this is a little early considering I still have some unwanted subcutaneous fat on my belly to go. I'll figure this out over the next day or two.

So that's it for today. I'm feeling so grateful that my body is allowing me to do the things that I thought were a thing of the past. I'm excited for the future. Gone are those days of guilt.

20 July 2020

Helvellyn

Helvellyn today and as I climbed the 3,162 ft elevation, then descended the 3,162 ft rocky paths, one thing kept coming to mind. This is getting easier. It is getting easier climbing up steep mountain sides. It is getting easier to keep going longer. Recovery is much quicker. I'm getting fit.

A super Monday, out with Jack and friend Alex today. The weather was a little gloomy with a few rain showers, but hey, we are mountain men. We don't melt in the rain, and we don't shrink either. Mountain climbing is exhilarating. The views, the fresh air, the sheer drops, the sound of silence. Simply wonderful.

I made a decision today to revisit the Yorkshire Three Peaks and push it as hard as I can. This will likely be a September visit to try and get some quiet up there and tackle the route in cooler weather. Our time stands at 11 hours and 53 minutes. I'm confident that with another couple of months training, a greater understanding of the challenge, and better weather, I can crack this in under 10 hours. A superb day.

21 July 2020

A good session this morning. 10km ran in 1 hour 8 minutes. This includes an elevation of over 600ft which slows me down as it's tough running up hills around here, but it's a milestone and now time to change from weight loss mode to athlete mode.

I'm going to switch from 22/23/24 fasts now to two lesser fasts per week. The fasts have done their job, exceeding all of my expectations by a mile, but now the concentration has to be on the daily level of exercise that I'm putting in. Thank you fasting!

Fitness is now back in the blood and I'm super excited at where this can take me. There are so many heavy challenges that I want to get do now. The National Three Peaks next week, if the Yorkshire marathon stays on, and I can get in, then I'll do it October 2020. The Manchester marathon is now April 2021, The Welsh 3000s, The Cairngorms 4000s, the coast to coast on the bike, and then an Ironman later in 2021.

This is so much better than eating rubbish and drinking booze every day. I look back and wonder why I did that to myself.

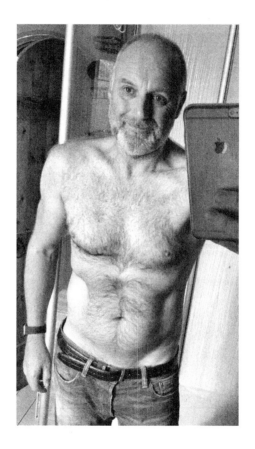

Target weight achieved!

24 July 2020

5 stone!

Done it! It is weigh-day and 5 whole stone of fat have gone. Goal achieved. I'm so happy. I'm 89.5kg.

I never thought this possible in four short months and it just shows what a sensible, consistent, informed strategy can do to a person's transformation. Proper nutrition, intermittent fasting, daily exercise, a reduction in stress, lots of water, and proper sleep.

I can honestly say that I have enjoyed every aspect of this transformation. I've enjoyed every meal, and I've had so much fun getting fit again. I've loved doing things that I've never done before. I've been the highest person in England. I've been the highest person in Wales. I love fitting back into favourite old clothes that were put away in the bottom of the wardrobe years ago. I've enjoyed buying new clothes several sizes smaller than I was. I've saved a fortune on the grocery bills. I've dropped so much guilt. I feel incredibly relaxed, and I feel 25 years younger. I'm so grateful.

Tonight Jack and I made the decision to book on a 10k run in November. We are doing this together which means a heck of a lot to me. As a lad and dad duo I really can't wait to get onto the start line together. This evening we started training together with an 8km run across the Pennines. It was fabulous to be able to train together. This transformation keeps on giving.

As I rode my bike this morning I was hurtling down a hill and looking across at the Pennine views. The sun was out and the air was fresh. I was totally invigorated by the experience. The thought crossed my mind back to pre-March when I'd get up, stressed, put the coffee machine on, and sit down with my laptop. What a difference! I really can't express how having the ability to do this stuff makes me feel. I just feel so young and fit.

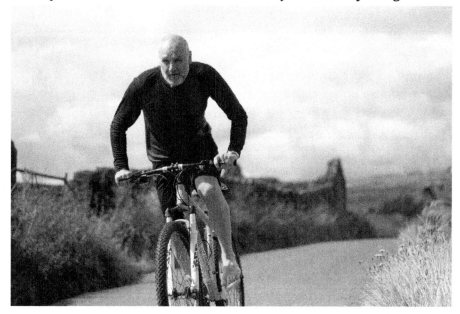

Out on my bike

In two days we're doing the National Three Peaks. We'll travel to Glasgow where we will meet Peter who is flying up. We'll stay over in the city and then travel to Fort William the next day. Around 6pm on Monday evening we start the ascend up Ben Nevis, followed by the drive and climb up Scafell Pike, followed by the drive and ascend up Snowdon. We have no doubt that we shall be totally shattered finishing up at Snowdon so we're going to book a hotel for that evening and have a few celebratory drinks and a nice meal. I can't wait.

28 July 2020

As I sit down to write this final journal entry of this wonderful journal I have to pay respect and deep appreciation to everyone who has supported me. I'm fit enough to move my body 25 miles and up and down 10,000ft of rocks, boulders, ditches, and rock faces across three countries in under 24 hours. If you are reading this then thank you for reading this far. If you have supported me on social media then I also thank you dearly.

The past couple of days have been a fantastic experience. Sunday morning started with a bike ride of around 10 miles to get my heart and legs going but without any impact to avoid potential injury. Packing my stuff and driving up to Glasgow, where we met Pete for a meal and a couple of drinks, was pretty cool. I felt alive and ready. A challenge whereby supporters had sponsored us for charity was now upon us. I am extremely grateful to everyone who committed their hard earned money for the generosity and trust they had placed in me to succeed.

We arrived in Glasgow and met up with Pete for a couple of beers and the first pizza in four months. I reckoned that as we would be exceeding over 85,000 steps a few carbs would be in order. I have to say, the fresh pizza tasted wonderful. The next morning we were up and out and driving to Fort William, the home of the highest mountain in Great Britain; Ben Nevis. We did a little sight-seeing on the way (Peter wasn't paying attention in the back seat and we were nearly in Oban before we realised!) and after stocking up on food in the local supermarket we were ready to go at 7.22pm.

Ben Nevis

The sky was heavy with dark cloud, and the rain had been coming and going all afternoon. Sadly at around 2000ft we entered cloud which wrecked the amazing mountain views that I had been looking forward to. But we weren't there for the views, we were there for the challenge. The start of the climb up Ben Nevis is tough from the Youth Hostel and a shock to the system. It's steep! It's really steep, but it's the fastest route we could have chosen and we wanted to be as quick as we could going up and then back down again. The reason for this speed is to limit the amount of time coming down in the pitch black over wet slippery rock with only head torches to help us see. On the way up, somewhere near 3,500ft, was a huge lump of snow. Snow in July! Incredible! After a couple of minutes taking photos, and throwing a few snowballs, we carefully packed the phones away and continue to press upwards.

As we reached the summit the wind was howling and the rain was driving into us horizontally. The light was drawing in fast, and wind chill felt like it was way below 0 degrees. The summit of Ben Nevis is rocky, we lost grass probably around 1000ft lower than the summit. We struggled across wet boulders until we hit the trail which was more of a shale type track. We high fived at the summit, took the obligatory photos and got off that mountain as quickly as we could. Feeling great, full of achievement for getting to the peak in great time, we ran downhill for a descent of possibly 2000ft until it was too dark and too dangerous to continue running. The next 2500ft or so was tricky as there were some pretty steep slopes and a lot of very slippery rocks. We eventually got back to the car after 3 hour and 35 minutes. We were cold and wet through and now it was down to Amanda to get us back to England and to Barrowdale, to hit Scafell Pike via the Corridor Route.

Scafell Pike

The journey south was clear and we made good time. The downside was that neither Pete or I managed to get any sleep. Only stopping en route once for two hot teas and a sparkling water for Amanda, we eventually arrived at Barrowdale at 4.40am. As we pulled up onto the farm's muddy wet field, the realisation that we had over four hours of hard climb in heavy rain, and in wet clothes, was extremely depressing. I have to say that at this point I just didn't want to put the wet hiking boots on and go. At 4.40am the night was still dark and it was cold. The next four hours was a killer and the summit was like something from another planet. Howling winds and freezing cold ice rain driving at us. It was impossible to speak to each other because of the wind. We had to get off the mountain as quickly as we could and back to the car for a change of clothes and some warmth. We arrived back at the car for 9.30am barely able to undo laces, zips and buttons due to frozen fingers.

Snowdon

Pete and I managed to grab a couple of hours sleep whilst Amanda drove to Wales and Snowdon. It's incredible that with only a couple of hours napping in a period of over 24 hours that the human body is capable of recovering from some pretty extreme exercise and be ready to go again. In our case, hiking and climbing to the summit of the highest mountain in Wales and back as fast as we could. Pete and I were delighted that the sun was now out having been drenched for hours. I had to put my wet through walking pants on, which was pretty horrible, but they soon dried in the mountain winds.

We managed to do Snowdon in 3 hours 21 minutes which resulted in a grand duration of 22 hours and 39 minutes for the whole of the Three Peaks Challenge. Coming back to meet Amanda, who was waiting for us with a big smile in the car park, felt absolutely fantastic. This was the conclusion to a 4 month journey that has seen my body, health, fitness, and wellbeing transform from a ticking health time bomb into somebody unrecognisable.

There have been so many well-wishers on social media who have congratulated me on all the hard work that I have put in to be able to complete challenges like this. Whilst I am ever so grateful for such wonderful comments, I have to say that it hasn't felt like hard work. It's been fun and I've thoroughly enjoyed the process. I've enjoyed every meal that I have eaten, I've loved getting out into the fresh air and moving, I loved seeing some amazing places on my mountain climbs, I've educated myself on nutrition, and I've made new friends.

Looking back on this journey it is difficult to say which aspect of change has been the biggest factor in this transformation. This is a question I'm asked a lot and if I had to choose one thing then it has to be the mindset to change. Without putting the head in the correct place then the change in nutrition, the fasting, the exercise, the hydration, the resting and relaxation, simply would not have happened.

Whilst not quite at the end of the book, this is my last journal entry. Phase one has changed my life. I know look forward to excitement of Phase 2. If you are starting your transformation then I wish you all the success in the world. Thanks for reading.

YOUR BODY IS
YOUR
GREATEST
ASSET

david

CHAPTER 8

The Weight-Loss Plateau

I thought it necessary to write about the weight-loss plateau towards the end of the book considering it is very likely that if you are going to carry out your own transformation then you are likely to hit your own plateau. As and when you hit yours don't worry, its normal. Whilst this is normal I would recommend having an understanding of why this occurs because when this happens it is too easy to get disillusioned and give up.

There are many reasons why a weight plateau will happen. These include:

Because you are losing fat and building muscle - just because the scales may not be changing, your shape is likely changing. Don't panic because in time the scales will continue to reflect the fat loss. This is just a gradual process that takes time.

Water retention masks fat loss - if you are not drinking enough water then your body will perceive this as a threat. It will hold onto what water it has. Without water, the kidneys can't function properly and they dump into the liver. As the liver is responsible for fat metabolism, it cannot work at optimal capacity. As a result, less fat gets metabolised, and your fat loss stalls. Drinking plenty of water helps you lose fat.

You are experiencing a period of re-adjustment - if you are stuck at the same weight for a few weeks, your body may just be at a reprogramming phase. The reason for this is that following all the changes the body is going through, you sometimes need to catch up. Just be patient because it will happen.

Your carbohydrate level is too high - many foods contain hidden carbohydrates. You may not realise it, but they could be creeping into your diet. You must consistently monitor your carb consumption as it could be too high. If you think this could be the case, you need to reconsider your food diary or ask a nutritionist to do it for you.

Your carbohydrate level is too low - if you are not eating enough carbs then your body will produce higher levels of adrenaline and cortisol. Clearly this can stall your weight loss. Your carbs should be coming from non-starchy vegetables, salads, and dark fruits like berries.

You are under-eating - a common pitfall. Not eating enough will result in your metabolism slowing down. Increase your consumption of healthy, whole food.

You aren't eating enough protein - if you aren't consuming enough protein, your body will break down its own protein (usually muscle) to create the energy it needs. Muscle loss will lower your metabolic rate.

You aren't exercising enough - whilst nutrition plays the biggest part in weight loss, not doing sufficient exercise can stall weight loss.

In relation to hitting a weight-loss plateau we should also be aware of hormonal levels. Hormones are the chemical messengers in the body that travel the bloodstream to the organs and tissues. An imbalance of hormones can lead to consistent weight gain over a long period of time, so losing those gains can prove to be very difficult. Important imbalances include:

Hypothyroidism - the thyroid is a small butterfly shaped gland in the neck, it manufactures hormones that control metabolism and growth. Weight gain can be affected when the thyroid produces too many or too few hormones. Hyperthyroidism (too many hormones) causes the metabolism to speed up, which can result in too much weight loss. Hypothyroidism (not enough hormone) results in a slower metabolism, which can cause weight gain.

Cortisol - stress affects the body in different ways. The three typical patterns are fight, flight, and defeat. Each pattern results in the secretion of different hormones. The defeat pattern creates a hormonal cascade that begins in the hypothalamus, in the brain, and results in cortisol secretion from the adrenal glands in the kidneys. It is cortisol that regulates energy production and mobilisation by selecting fat, protein or carbohydrates. When cortisol production is high, it can increase a person's cravings for sugar and fat, as well as increasing the appetite generally, which can cause weight gain.

Food intolerances - An intolerance is the difficulty of digesting certain foods and having an unpleasant physical reaction to them. It can cause symptoms, such as bloating and stomach pain, which usually happen a few hours after eating the food.

Whilst any food can cause an intolerance, the most common foods to cause an intolerance are milk, wheat, eggs, yeast and nuts. According to Cambridge Nutritional Sciences, 40% of their clients tested positive to dairy. Wheat accounted for about 25% of all food intolerances.

Food intolerances are linked to weight gain because it is common to crave foods that we are intolerant to. An estimated 50% of people with a food intolerance crave the food that their bodies can't handle. If we don't consume these foods, then withdrawal symptoms may kick in and this often results in binge eating and weight gain.

Food intolerances can also give you low energy. The effort involved in processing a food that you are intolerant to can put a strain on your system. This can cause low energy levels which can lead to a person becoming less active, which in turn can result in weight gain.

CHAPTER 9

*My Blueprint to Health, Fitness,
and Wellbeing*

I n business it is absolutely essential to systemise the operations enough so that the people within that business can work to a proven blueprint or plan to achieve the desired success.

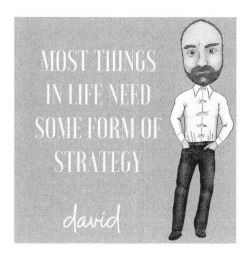

MOST THINGS
IN LIFE NEED
SOME FORM OF
STRATEGY

david

When regaining our health and wellbeing, there are a number of factors that must be aligned to succeed and maintain that success. I believe therefore, that it is essential that we work to a system. With this in mind I have integrated all the elements of goal setting, mindset, nutrition, fasting, and exercise into what I call The Fit4Business Blueprint.

As mentioned earlier in the book, there are so many contradictory ideas by so called experts (many of whom have a commercial agenda) which ultimately lead most of us to fail. It is hardly surprising that there is such an obesity problem, with such a huge percentage of the world's populations, which often results in chronic illness and premature death.

The Fit4Business Blueprint is an easy to follow step by step process on how I achieved my 70lb weight loss and return to fitness so quickly, and so effectively.

1. The Personal Purpose Plan™

This module explores your current position in terms of health, fitness, and nutrition. We look at the demands on your available time and any challenges that are affecting your lifestyle. When these elements have been explored thoroughly we plan where you need to, or want to, be including weight, fitness, and lifestyle.

2. The Motivated Mindset Matrix™

This module looks at what has made us get to where we are now? What will get us to where we want to be in the future? What is it that we want? What will keep us in that brilliant new state for the long term? Mindset is critical and if we are to change our lives for the better then we need put ourselves in an absolute state of certainty.

3. The Natural Nutrition Network™

We know that there is an incredible amount of confusing contradictions out there. We also know that if we don't adopt a healthy and sustainable plan then we are bound to fail. This doesn't have to be complicated. In fact complicated often equals failure. I set out my own plan and I have loved and enjoyed every meal I have eaten without ever feeling as though I'm dieting or depriving myself. I don't want to live my life counting calories, and I'm sure you don't want to too.

4. The Free Fasting Formula™

A huge aspect of my health transformation explained in detail. Nutrition is crucial but so are meal times and knowing the best time to exercise. Get this right and accelerate your results. Schedule more time time back into your life, and save £thousands.

5. The Easy Exercise Explainer™

It is no surprise at all that people join a gym at the start of January, and then give up by the start of February. Exercise has to suit you, your current situation, your goals, and most of all you have to love it. Exercise should be fun and rewarding, not something to dread.

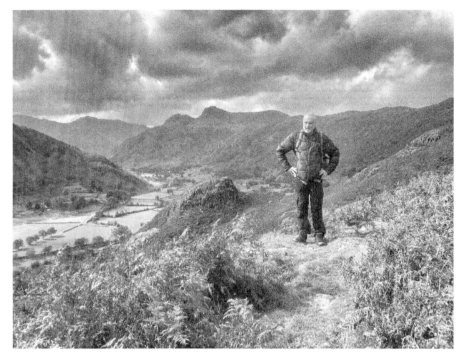

*Climbing up Bowness, Lake District, in September
2020 at 13st 10lbs (87.7kg)*

If you are interested in working with me then please visit my website **www.davefernley.com** and drop me a note.

I blog on the website every couple of days with new things that I am doing, and learning, on my own journey. I hope to connect with you.

We also have a growing Facebook group - Fit For Business - full of people actively engaging with their health and supporting each other.

If you are interested in joining our monthly subscription programme or our premium packages including health and wellness retreats and climbing challenges, please contact me through my website, or Facebook.

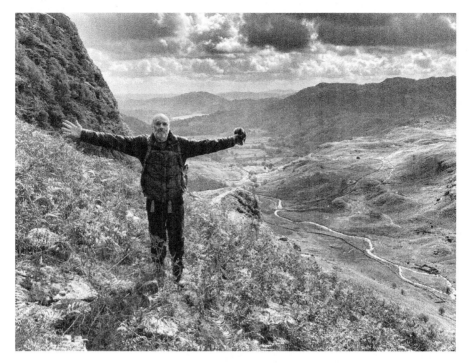

Climbing up Bowness, Lake District, in September 2020 at 13st 10lbs (87.7kg)

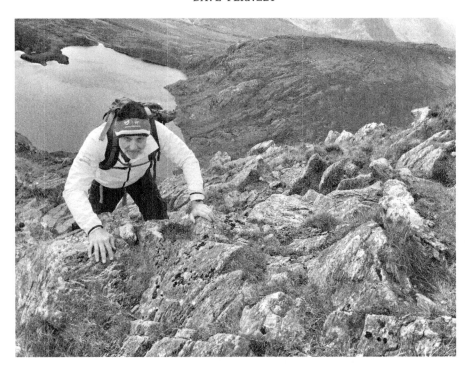

I'm currently training as a Mountain Leader, so that I can lead groups of people who also want to achieve a state of health and fitness.

AND FINALLY

I've loved writing this book and if you have read to this point I want to thank you for showing an interest in what I have done. I sincerely hope that if you are setting out on your own transformation, you are able to make the necessary changes to get your greatest asset into a place where you can live an amazing and fulfilled life.

It is absolutely my intention to write a second book which will cover the next phase of my progression. I'm already excited to explore what a fat middle aged, stressed up, bloke who drank too much and ate too much rubbish, can do. I look forward to running a marathon. I have just registered for the Hell of a Hill Marathon in November. I look forward to increasing the mountain adventures, and I look forward to doing lots of other challenges such as the coast to coast bike ride and the Brutal Triathlon in Snowdonia next year.

I also look forward to developing my knowledge in the field of nutrition, fitness, health, and wellbeing. Having now obtained an Diet and Nutritional Advisor Diploma, an Advanced Nutrition for Weight Loss Diploma, and an NLP Practitioner Diploma, I am finding the whole learning experience fascinating. Having already been a trainer and mentor in property for a number of years, this is an area that I am extremely interested in. I fully intend to continue my development in this area.

I also look forward to working with people who are making the all-important changes in their lives to gain health and fitness. Having spoken to many people over the years, and particularly during my transformation, it seems clear to me that so many people, and I include myself, have been taught lessons which only set them up to fail. It's a dreadful situation that people are becoming ill, and are dying, as a consequence of wrong information, some of which is purely for commercial gain. It is my intention to run some retreats and some other really cool programmes for people who want to make some transformations and want me to help them.

The past four months has been incredible. I've walked up mountains, ran, jumped on bikes for the first time in probably 30 years, walked away from the XXXL rail and towards the M rail, connected with my kids again through new activity, saved myself a fortune on booze, take outs, and junk food, and received the most amazing messages from people that I know, and people that I have never met. I've cured symptoms that have plagued me for years like indigestion, reflux, sleep apnea, snoring, cracked feet, and constant colds and flu.

I've had lots of people say how much younger I look. I can tell you that I feel younger. I feel 30 again. I'm more relaxed. I'm more focused. I'm more appreciative of life. If you are wanting to make your transformation, however you do it, always remember to have fun.

Be strong

David

PS This is my first book. I'm not a reader and I've never been into books, so it amazes me that I have even managed to write one. I still can't quite believe that I will be publishing it for sale!

I've been blown away by the messages of support in my inbox and truly touched. I've really enjoyed hearing from people who have comment, liked, or shared my posts and travelled my weight loss journey with me.

My journey continues so I have started to jot down some notes for my next book which is all about the challenges I am signing myself up for, marathons and triathlons (assuming they will ever happen again) and becoming a fully trained and insured Mountain Leader. I also need to keep this weight off, and not slide slowly back to 19 stone.

It's a researched fact that people will read reviews before buying a book, and many people won't buy a book if there are no reviews.

If you have got anything from my book, or think someone else will, please leave a review. This will really help me, and my book, and give me the momentum to carry on doing what doesn't come naturally to me. Writing! :o)

CONTACT

You can find me in various places on the internet:

Facebook - David Fernley

Facebook Page - Fit for Business with David Fernley

Facebook Group - Fit for Business

Linkedin - David Fernley FCMI

Instagram - fernleydavid

Website - DaveFernley.com

Twitter - David Fernley

Book - 5 Stone, 4 Months, 3 Mountains

Email - david@clarusproperties

I'd love to hear from you.

ABOUT THE AUTHOR

Dave Fernley

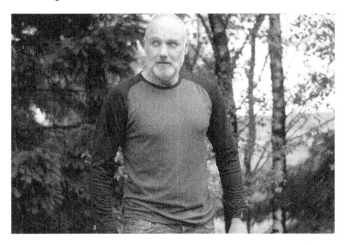

Entrepreneur Dave Fernley was three months away from his 50th birthday when the UK went into Lockdown because of Covid-19. His property training business faced ruin as every planned and prepared for event had to be cancelled and all delegates refunded. With business and income falling apart, and with no end in sight, Dave had no control over anything anymore.

Except one thing. His health and fitness. Stress from an acrimonious divorce, family court matters, and running several businesses had seen Dave's weight increase to just over 19 stone. Now or never, he decided to get healthy and fit again using just good food and the countryside.

Dave has documented his journey on Facebook and Instagram sharing his shame and his determination - to recover his health and body - with family and friends. Within just 4 months, he lost an astonishing 5 stone, without supplements, gyms, surgery, calorie counting, or a personal trainer.

Here, for the first time, Dave shares his story, tips, and recipes, to show how you don't need to spend a lot of money, or need a lot of time to get healthy. At a now fit and healthy 13st 12lb he is now climbing mountains, regularly running 10 miles a day, as well as training for marathons and triathlons.

After such an astonishing transformation, Dave is now helping other business people to achieve their own health and fitness transformations through a structured programme. Now training as a Mountain Leader he is teaching others to appreciate our countryside as a natural stress reliever and health provider.

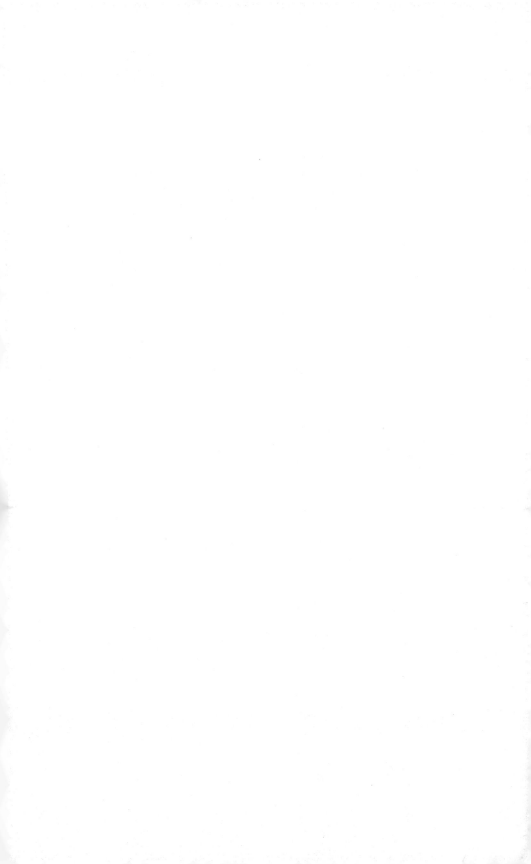

Printed in Great Britain
by Amazon

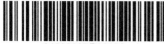